PSYCHOTHERAPIST'S RESOURCE ON PSYCHIATRIC MEDICATIONS

D0094352

www.wadsworth.com

wadsworth.com is the World Wide Web site for Wadsworth
and is your direct source to dozens of online resources.

At *wadsworth.com* you can find out about
supplements, demonstration software, and
student resources. You can also send e-mail to many of our
authors and preview new publications and exciting new
technologies.

wadsworth.com
Changing the way the world learns®

Mary M. Clarkson

PSYCHOTHERAPIST'S RESOURCE ON
PSYCHIATRIC MEDICATIONS

ISSUES OF TREATMENT AND REFERRAL

GEORGE BUELOW

University of Southern Mississippi

SUZANNE HEBERT

University of Mississippi

SIDNE BUELOW

Pine Belt Mental Health Resources

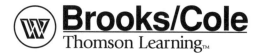

Australia • Canada • Denmark • Japan • Mexico • New Zealand • Philippines
Puerto Rico • Singapore • South Africa • Spain • United Kingdom • United States

Counseling Editor: Eileen Murphy
Assistant Editor: Julie Martinez
Editorial Assistant: Annie Berterretche
Marketing Manager: Joanne Terhaar
Marketing Assistant: Jenna Burrill
Project Editor: Tanya Nigh
Print Buyer: Mary Noel
Permissions Editor: Joohee Lee
Production Service: Progressive
   Information Technologies

Text Designer: Laurie Albrecht
Copy Editor: Progressive Publishing
   Alternatives
Compositor: Progressive Information
   Technologies
Cover Designer: Bill Stanton
Cover Printer: Webcom Limited
Printer/Binder: Webcom Limited

Printed in Canada
      5   6   7   03

For permission to use material from
this text, contact us:
   Web: www.thomsonrights.com
   Fax: 1-800-730-2215
   Phone: 1-800-730-2214

ISBN: 0-534-35703-2

For more information, contact
Wadsworth/Thomson Learning
10 Davis Drive
Belmont, CA 94002-3098
USA
www.wadsworth.com

International Headquarters
Thomson Learning
290 Harbor Drive, 2nd Floor
Stamford, CT 06902-7477
USA

UK/Europe/Middle East
Thomson Learning
Berkshire House
168-173 High Holborn
London WC1V 7AA
United Kingdom

Asia
Thomson Learning
60 Albert Street #15-01
Albert Complex
Singapore 189969

Canada
Nelson/Thomson Learning
1120 Birchmount Road
Scarborough, Ontario M1K 5G4
Canada

Contents

PREFACE

This book is an introduction for psychotherapists to the treatment and referral issues that surround commonly prescribed psychiatric drugs. It provides an overview of psychopharmacology as it affects therapists' work with clients who are already using psychiatric medications or who potentially should be. This book provides up-to-date information on the mechanisms of action and side effects of typically prescribed psychiatric medications, including antidepressants, antianxiety agents, antipsychotics, and pain medications. It is not meant to be exhaustive in every area of practice, and therapists should keep abreast of the latest psychopharmacology journals to access current information on the most current psychiatric medications.

Because of the recent explosion of knowledge through biochemistry research, psychopharmacology texts have become difficult for many therapists to read and fully understand. Even so, therapists often work with clients who are taking psychiatric medications with which neither client nor therapist is familiar. Not only are therapists faced with a wide range of medications, but they also are often at a loss about how to work with prescribing physicians. In addition, many therapists do not know whether or how to work on medical-compliance issues as central concerns in therapy. Contemporary jobs in counseling, psychiatric nursing, social work, family therapy, and psychology, both in private and public practice, require a clear understanding of pharmacopsychological issues. We define pharmacopsychological issues as those within the scope of practice of psychologists who are being trained to prescribe psychiatric drugs.

We wrote this book as (a) an introductory text for those studying drugs used in treating mental illness; (b) a reference for advanced undergraduate and graduate students in counseling, guidance, nursing, social work, and psychology; and (c) a resource for therapists and practitioners who work in the field and often have only the *Physicians' Desk Reference* (PDR) as a guide to understanding the psychiatric drugs used by their clients. In *Psychotherapist's Resource on Psychiatric Medications*, each chapter is meant to stand alone so that, without having to review other chapters, readers can refer to a particular diagnostic area, the drugs most frequently used, their usual actions, and their side effects.

This book is organized under headings that are familiar to clinicians. It begins with an introductory chapter in which we examine treatment and referral issues that therapists face when working with clients, and provide information about the processes of neurotransmission. Then, in Chapters 2 through 5, we discuss the major psychiatric disorders for which clients are most likely to be using psychiatric drugs, including: depression and manic-depression, anxiety and panic disorders, psychosis, and pain. We included the chapter on pain because chronic pain usually has both a physical and psychogenic side and because pain medications often produce psychiatric effects.

Chapters 2 through 5 each begin with an introduction to the etiology of a specific psychiatric problem, followed by a discussion of the mechanisms of action for the classes of drugs used to treat the problem, so that therapists can better understand the medical intention of the drugs. In these chapters, we discuss the most common drug treatments, drug and therapy interaction, and referral issues that arise within a specific diagnostic area. Throughout this book, we emphasize the need for an understanding of how various drugs influence the workings of the nervous system through neurotransmission and, thus, the symptomatology of the psychiatric disorder.

To assist readers further, we have included Appendix A briefly describing the central nervous system as well as a glossary.

ACKNOWLEDGEMENTS

We wish to acknowledge the people whose support, encouragement, and suggestions have helped us in writing this book. First, we want to thank those who reviewed earlier versions of the manuscript, including Thomas McGovern, Texas Tech Health Sciences Center; Dorothy Neufeld, Loma Linda University; and Howard J. Shaffer, Harvard Medical School-The Cambridge Hospital.

We would also like to thank the staff at Brooks/Cole, especially Eileen Murphy and Julie Martinez for their assistance in developing and publishing this book.

George Buelow
Suzanne Hebert
Sidne Buelow

1

PART 1: PSYCHOTHERAPISTS AND PSYCHIATRIC MEDICINES

Client referral to psychiatrists or family physicians for evaluation of the appropriateness of psychiatric medication causes a strong emotional reaction for many psychotherapists. When asked if they feel comfortable making referrals for psychiatric drug intervention, a significant minority of graduate therapists respond that they don't believe people should use drugs for emotional problems, especially for anxiety and depression. As the issue is debated in class, salient features of therapists' beliefs about drugs, usually in the absence of course work in pharmacopsychology, are that (a) drugs should be a last resort and should be used primarily to treat psychoses (schizophrenia, for example); (b) psychiatric drugs do not differ a great deal from recreational drugs people use to relieve boredom or depression (cocaine, for example) or anxiety (alcohol and narcotics, for example); (c) such a wide gulf exists between psychotherapists and psychiatrists that communication is difficult or impossible; (d) learning about psychiatric drugs is difficult and working with clients who are on psychiatric drugs, or referring them, will raise counselors' malpractice liability; and (e) drugs cannot cure mental illnesses and, thus, are not superior to psychotherapy or even to a placebo. Unfortunately, this belief system, which comes less from experience than from family and societal values, is often shared by the therapists and the clients they see.

Due to the lack of emphasis on biopsychological training in counseling, family therapy, social work, nursing, and psychology programs, many therapists are not prepared in pharmacopsychology, the study of psychoactive medications. The belief systems therapists hold often inhibit them from gaining practical experience in this important area. These irrational beliefs are often reinforced by the limited educational opportunities available that could provide insight and encourage practical experience. Lack of preparation has slowed the development of the field of psychotherapy in two ways. First, at the individual level, it has hindered therapists' effectiveness in working with clients who are taking psychiatric medications and has impeded referral of clients who need both psychiatric medications and psychotherapy. Second, at the professional level, therapists' lack of expertise in this rapidly developing area negatively reflects on the stature of psychotherapy as a force within the competitive community of health care providers. Lack of expertise also presents ethical problems. It is unethical to work with clients using traditional psychotherapy techniques alone when a great deal of suffering could be alleviated, and the therapy process could itself be enhanced, by judicious use of psychiatric medications.

Finally, legal problems may well emerge if therapists are not both informed and prudent in their decisions to treat and refer clients who are in need of psychiatric medications. The liability incurred in not referring a client for appraisal of need for psychiatric medication is certainly much higher than referring a client who does not. Good faith client referral is the therapists' responsibility; the decision to prescribe rests with the psychiatrist or family physician.

Today, therapists are trained to work with an increasingly more difficult client population. In community mental health centers, chemical dependence treatment programs, college counseling centers, and private practice, therapists face a variety of difficult and complex psychiatric cases. National certification requires that therapists, especially counselors and psychologists, be trained to provide expertise in developmental deficiencies, crisis intervention, remediation of emotional problems, couples and family therapy, accurate appraisal and assessment, and consultation within the community. Psychiatric medications may be in use in any one of these settings. For example, psychotherapists assess and work with children who have been diagnosed as having attention deficit disorder with hyperactivity (ADHD). Many ADHD diagnosed children may have been taking methylphenidate (Ritalin) for various periods of time with varying therapeutic results. Individuals in crisis, whom therapists commonly see in a variety of community mental health and hospital settings, have often been prescribed tranquilizers or sedative hypnotic agents (such as Xanax or Valium) without adequate psychological assessment. Finally, even if certification and licensure for psychotherapists and psychologists did not support development of expertise in these areas, the pragmatics of both public and private practice certainly would. Knowledge of the use of psychiatric medications is clearly becoming a necessary step in the development of the science and art of psychotherapy.

This book is designed to provide up-to-date information on what therapists have traditionally been expected to know, such as support for drug compliance. However, it also provides a firm base in areas that practitioners are increasingly confronting, such as the neuropharmacology of typically prescribed psychiatric medications. Regardless of where you stand on the issues, future counseling and clinical psychologists, as psychiatric health care providers with hospital privileges, may well be expected to know psychiatric medications well enough to prescribe them! Pharmacopsychologists are already being trained to prescribe in national and state-sponsored postdoctoral programs.

REFERRAL ISSUES

Perhaps as challenging as working with clients on medication issues, psychotherapists must learn to talk effectively with physicians about the efficacy and side effects of prescribed medications, as well as compliance problems following referral. Therapists must also establish good working relationships with physicians, including psychiatrists, in the local community so they can effectively refer their clients and monitor compliance when necessary. The referral picture is complicated by the fact that approximately 70% of antianxiety and antidepressant drugs are prescribed by family physicians and other doctors not extensively trained in psychiatry.

Two of the most frequently prescribed medications, benzodiazepines (antianxiety agents such as Xanax) and fluoxetine (Prozac for depression), are usually not lethal in suicide attempts when taken in moderate doses or alone (without other drugs to potentiate them or increase their actions). Thus, family physicians feel, perhaps unwisely, at lower risk in prescribing them. Further, because psychiatrists' office charges are often more expensive than a visit to a family physician, patients quite reasonably are more likely to choose the latter. Finally, because an onus exists on visiting a psychiatrist, patients are more likely to go to their family physician initially for depression or anxiety.

Many physicians are not as aware of the benefits of psychotherapy for their patients as they need to be. Although the picture is changing rapidly, many physicians do not commonly refer patients for psychotherapy services in the community or utilize feedback from mental health workers as effectively as they should. It is necessary, therefore, for therapists to help structure meaningful dialogue with psychiatrists and family physicians in their communities about patient medications and about the value of concurrent psychotherapy. Case studies in subsequent chapters will discuss these concerns.

Even though therapists are not responsible for med-checks, physicians need independent feedback on their patient's social adaptation, mental status, physical functioning, and medication compliance. Examples of specific information that should be related to physicians by therapists are:

- reported changes in sleep or eating habits
- reported changes in amount of social contacts, activities, and work or school attendance
- reported feeling state (such as sad, depressed, angry)
- observed mood state (such as anxious, depressed, euphoric, or labile)
- evidence of psychotic behaviors (delusions or hallucinations)
- evidence of suicidal or homicidal ideation or behaviors
- observed physical movement activity (psychomotor agitation or retardation)

Often, patients spend more time with their counselors than their physicians, which can provide therapists greater opportunities to obtain this important information.

Like psychotherapists, physicians want and need feedback that is accurate, specific, and timely. It is best, therefore, to have the most salient issues written down and the chart available before contacting a client's physician by phone. Phone contacts should be followed up in writing so specifics of the conversation are reflected in the written record. If clear liaisons are built in a personal way, many physicians are willing to see clients to evaluate them for possible psychiatric medication on the recommendation and referral of counselors and other psychotherapists. To provide information on request to a physician or to initiate any contact on the client's behalf, therapists must remember to have clients provide written consent. When making referrals for medication evaluation, for example, even in cases where the client has chosen his or her family physician to do the evaluation, it is important to first obtain a written consent from the client before contacting and forwarding records to the nurse case-managers and to the physician. A letter should be sent to the physician at that time outlining the specific symptoms that initiated the referral. Psychological judgments and interpretations should be kept to a minimum, and psychological jargon should not be used. As a general rule, clients should be referred to a psychiatrist or practitioner with prescription privileges for evaluation for medication or inpatient treatment under the following conditions:

- when they are no longer benefiting from psychotherapy because they are too depressed to take consistent action to make cognitive, affective, and behavioral changes or so manic that their judgment is becoming unsound
- when they are too anxious to make progress using proven anxiety management techniques
- when their cognitions are loosely enough connected to confuse you, even after having established a therapeutic alliance
- when they are a high or rising suicide risk
- when they are dual-diagnosis clients and they have relapsed back into alcohol or other drug use

In a clinical practice, therapists often face situations where a client has been taking a medication that was prescribed by the family doctor and their symptomatology does not improve or even worsens. The therapist is expected to communicate this valuable information to the client's prescribing physician. Unfortunately, there are times that a client does not improve even after the doctor has appropriately responded by adjusting the dose and/or prescribing a different medication. The therapist should discuss observations and the option of a referral to a psychiatrist with the client. Considering boundary issues regarding physicians' clientele and the desirability of mental health professionals' maintaining good relationships with the doctors in their community, caution must be exercised in exploring the need for referral to a psychiatrist.

Symptoms or other situations that warrant a recommendation to a psychiatrist are:

- evidence of psychotic behavior
- current suicidal or homicidal ideation, especially if a history of impulsive or harmful behaviors is present
- current intrusive and severe symptoms of PTSD
- current intrusive and severe symptoms of an eating disorder
- significant symptoms for the diagnosis of more than one DSM-IV Axis I psychiatric disorder (i.e., concurrent symptoms of obsessive-compulsive disorder with major depression)
- episode of major depression with severe symptomatology and history of suicide attempts
- dissociative identity disorder with suicidal or homicidal ideation
- panic disorder with agoraphobia

Once the decision has been made to refer a client to a psychiatrist, the therapist should organize pertinent information regarding the client in the form of a referral letter. Below is an example of a referral letter to a psychiatrist.

RE: Referral of Julie D.
SS# 000 00 000
Dear Dr. Smith,

The purpose of this correspondence is to provide information on a client who has been referred to you. Julie D. is a 22-year-old single Caucasian female. She has completed three years of college and plans to return to school. However, at this time, she is working in a department store on a full-time basis. Her family resides out of state, and she lives with two roommates in an apartment in town.

Julie began therapy at Willow Place Outpatient Counseling Center in May of 1997. To date, she has attended a total of 16 therapy sessions. Based on her report, this is her first treatment episode with a mental health professional. She has been compliant in therapy and has demonstrated a willingness to get better.

Continued

Julie has been treated under the diagnosis of major depression. Initially, she presented with symptoms of depressed mood, excessive worrying, loss of interest in her activities, irritability, interrupted sleep, extreme fatigue, psychomotor agitation, low self-esteem, and problems concentrating. Two weeks ago, she disclosed that she has been binging and purging at a rate of about three times a week. Julie indicated that these symptoms began about six weeks ago. Exploration revealed that she last experienced these eating-disorder symptoms in her last semester of college and dropped out of school because she "feared others would discover what I was doing."

I would appreciate you performing a psychiatric evaluation and assessing Julie for the appropriateness of drug therapy. Although Julie has expressed fear about seeing a psychiatrist, I think you will experience her as a pleasant individual. I look forward to receiving your evaluation and recommendations for treatment. Your time, energy and expertise are appreciated.
Sincerely,

When the client signs a release for you to contact a physician, recall that it may speed up the process to attach an original signed consent form from the client allowing the physician to communicate his or her findings to you. Remember to retain a copy for your files.

Clients make slow or no progress in psychotherapy for a multitude of reasons. However, therapists (and certainly clients) often misinterpret why they seem stuck in therapy. Therefore, therapy should be continually reevaluated to determine whether clients are resistant or malingering, whether the therapist is using the wrong techniques, or whether clients' lack of progress is caused by underlying neuropsychological problems that medications might well reduce. Our experience clearly indicates that many therapists see psychiatric medications as a last resort for failed therapy rather than as a complement to therapy. If psychotherapists do not learn the basics of pharmacopsychology and the actions of modern psychiatric drugs, this view will not change. Further, many chemical dependence therapists fear that psychotropic medications constitute another source of abusable chemicals that will negatively impact clients' recovery. On the contrary, clients who need and take prescribed psychotropic medication are at lower risk for relapse.

A physician may ask the therapist for a recommendation on a drug to be prescribed, or a therapist may inadvertently offer such advice by referring the patient for an antidepressant rather than for an evaluation for depression. Therapists should decline to make such recommendations unless they are specifically trained as pharmacy consultants because they would be operating beyond the scope of their expertise. Physicians routinely include summaries of such advice in the patient's record, summaries that may serve to establish a legal bridge to the therapist if the patient suffers harm from a specifically discussed medication.

By gaining knowledge in the field of pharmacopsychology, therapists learn that one drug can have many uses or indications. For example, a client who is prescribed an antidepressant medication, such as Elavil, may not be depressed but may have been prescribed an antidepressant for chronic pain; Chapter 2 enumerates other uses for antidepressant drugs. Pharmaceutical companies not only introduce new drugs into the market but they also invest their resources testing new uses for established drugs. Therapists familiar with appropriate uses for particular medications are not as likely to mistakenly assume why a client is prescribed a particular drug.

Finally, it must be emphasized that psychiatric medications are not a magic bullet. They do not simply go to the center of the problem and destroy it. Medications reach throughout the body and affect most of its systems. Side effects are the product of this lack of specificity. Psychiatric medications do not exactly imitate the neurotransmitters whose actions they were designed to mimic and may produce other, though usually less severe, psychiatric symptoms. Further, individuals respond very differently to different drugs and different levels of drugs. Both drug and dose must fit the patient. During the early adjustment period, while side effects are most evident, medication management between physician and patient is most fragile. It is during this period of change that clients need the most support and therapists need the most expertise. Likewise, it is during periods of disciplinary change that therapists have the most difficulty coping with new directions in their field. This book is designed to facilitate movement through this developmental period not only with clients but also within the psychotherapy discipline itself as pharmacopsychology takes its place as a necessary area of study.

1. Referral reasons
2. Know side-effects
3. Drug compliance
4. Drug psychoeducation

TREATMENT ISSUES

Psychotherapists are routinely faced with a number of converging problems with clients' use of psychiatric medications. First, therapists are expected to know the conditions under which clients should be referred to a physician for appraisal for medication. Second, therapists are expected to understand the experience and side-effect problems clients have with their medications. Third, therapists are expected to help clients with drug compliance. Fourth, psychotherapists are expected to educate clients about the interactions of their psychiatric medications and alcohol or illicit drugs and to understand issues of dual diagnosis. A useful understanding of each of these areas presupposes a general knowledge of pharmacopsychology, including neurotransmitters and drug interactions as well as specific knowledge of frequently prescribed antidepressant, antianxiety, and antipsychotic medications.

FACTORS THAT IMPACT EFFECTIVENESS OF PRESCRIBED MEDICATIONS

Numerous factors influence medication effects on the human body. Elements such as patient compliance and medication form (i.e., intravenous or oral formulation), have direct consequences, whereas other social and economic influences indirectly impact the availability of medication for patients.

ECONOMIC AND SOCIAL FACTORS

Historically, mental health care expenses have been reimbursed by health insurers at a significantly lower rate than physical health care problems. Typically, insurance companies cover 80% of physical health problems, such as heart or cardiovascular diseases. It is common, however, for visits to mental health care facilities to be reimbursed at only 50%. Further, total lifetime benefits (or cap) for mental health diagnoses are often set by an insurance company at a much lower level. For example, XYZ Insurance Company's schedule of benefits may provide a lifetime maximum benefit of $1,000,000 for physical conditions, but for nervous/mental conditions, the lifetime maximum benefit is reduced to $15,000. Recently, the issue of parity has been addressed by state and federal legislative bodies throughout the United States. Some progress has been made. Laws passed in a variety of states address this issue in an effort to decrease the disparity, and, the Federal Mental Health Parity Act went into effect in January of 1988. The purpose of this legislation was to help eliminate discrimination against people with mental health problems. However, there are significant mental health-related exclusions that limit the new law's ability to affect needed changes (Ziegler, 1997).

Despite the fact that the new parity legislation may increase coverage for mental health care illnesses, a new force, managed care, has already impacted health care reimbursements. The evolution of managed care was precipitated by rapidly rising health care costs over the last several decades and by economic incentives for companies who had previously been institutional middlemen in the health care fields, particularly insurance companies. In the mental health arena, managed care works by closely regulating and/or restricting the number and type of services (or visits) to therapists and hospitals. Interestingly, managed care companies often provide disproportionate support for inpatient versus outpatient treatment. The reduction in the number of counseling and psychotherapy sessions for which insurance may be billed has led to a greater reliance on prescription medication. Thus, a challenge arises for individuals with chronic mental health problems and their attending therapists and doctors. Mental health services for needy individuals cannot exist in the absence of monitoring outcomes or considering alternatives, particularly psychiatric medications. Therapists must consider these alternatives as an adjunct to their therapy interventions, and must track their effectiveness in the recovery and stabilization of individuals with serious and persistent mental illnesses. Note that managed care companies have incorrectly disseminated the view that therapists as a group have done a less-than-adequate job of monitoring clients' time in treatment. For selected groups of clients, more time in treatment is associated with more stable improvement.

CLIENTS' RESPONSIBILITY

Managed care dictates that mental health care workers change how they provide services to their patients. More emphasis must be placed on clients' responsibility and on better determining what clients can do to help themselves. Therapists can assist clients by imparting knowledge regarding behavioral steps that will augment their medications' therapeutic effects and lead to further empowerment.

For example, Glen, a 48-year-old male reported that he had been "sick" most of his adult life. At the age of 20, Glen was a bright young man attending college when his illness surfaced. Over several years, and after repeated hospitalization, Glen was diagnosed with paranoid schizophrenia. He explained that he had tried to work but continued to fail in life due to relapses of his mental illness. After more than a decade of frustration, he began attending groups that helped him gain knowledge about his disease and that involved his family in a more positive way. Glen indicated that an in-depth knowledge of schizophrenia and the medications used to treat it assisted him in developing more realistic self-expectations, decreasing self-blame, increasing his self-acceptance, and helping him better utilize his family's resources. He has become more compliant with his medication regime, more accepting of side effects, and gradually stopped recreational drinking. Also, Glen reported that he learned the warning signs of relapse and what behaviors increase his relapse risk. He learned how to talk more openly with his doctor. During the past several years, Glen has been hospitalized much less frequently. In this case, family and individual education helped decrease embarrassment, shame, and guilt about Glen's mental condition. Understanding the biological basis of the disease and how psychiatric medications help control symptoms assisted Glen in decreasing the number of exacerbations (breakthroughs) of the illness and become better able to manage his medications. With appropriate knowledge, clients are better equipped to make decisions regarding their wellbeing, which leads in turn to improvements in functioning and decreases in health care costs.

In addition to education about specific mental illness, therapists can increase clients' awareness of the daily choices made about eating, sleeping, activity levels, and alcohol and drug use. Behaviors that affect the body's metabolism affect a drug's effectiveness. Therapists can serve their clients better by actively promoting a wellness model that endorses a holistic approach to recovery. For example, people who quit smoking often do so on the advice of a health professional. Recommendations for a healthy lifestyle must be supported by the counselor's emphasis on these areas, including: (1) balanced

diet; (2) appropriate amount and type of exercise; (3) avoidance of alcohol, tobacco, and unprescribed drugs; (4) avoidance of caffeine; (5) adequate rest and
sleep; and (6) a reasonable balance between work and leisure activities.

Therapists working with clients in settings where the length of therapy
session is longer than an hour (such as inpatient, partial hospital, or intensive
outpatient groups) have greater opportunities to observe clients' behaviors.
DeFreita and Swartz (1979) indicate, for example, that by increasing the intake
of caffeine, patients often initiate a cycle of increasing anxiety and irritability
leading to higher dosage of prescription medications with sedative characteristics. Without an awareness of or education on caffeine's effects, this vicious
cycle can develop and greatly complicate both medical (e.g., blood pressure
fluctuations) and psychiatric problems. Consider the case of Zeke, a 34-year-
old white single male, who had decompensated after attending individual
therapy for 3 months. Zeke's psychiatrist had avoided placing him in a more
intensive level of therapy by increasing the dose of an antidepressant, Zoloft,
and prescribing another antidepressant, trazadone (Deseryl), for sleep. Despite
appropriate attention and treatment from his psychiatrist, Zeke required more
intensive treatment in a partial hospital program. Therapists in the program
noted that Zeke consumed many caffeinated beverages, which he said helped
him stay awake. Further investigation of Zeke's situation revealed that he was
drinking caffeinated soft drinks and coffee throughout the day to counter the
sedative effects of his psychiatric medications.

Although most people consume caffeinated drinks for their stimulating effects, caffeine has numerous other effects on the body, including insomnia, excitement, nervousness, ringing in the ears, headaches, lightheadedness, increased urination, increased heart rate, nausea, vomiting, and diarrhea (Olin et
al., 1998). Caffeine's cluster of effects resembles symptoms of anxiety disorders. Therefore, clients with anxiety problems (which are often associated with
depression) need to be reminded that they can help themselves by avoiding
caffeine. By learning the caffeine content in a variety of drinks, therapists can
educate clients on possible outcomes of their choices. The following table illustrates the variation of caffeine content in drinks.

Comparison of Caffeine Contents:

Regular brewed coffee	40–180 mg per 5–8 ounces
Regular instant coffee	30–120 mg per 5–8 ounces
Decaffeinated brewed coffee	2.5 mg per 5–8 ounces
Decaffeinated instant coffee	1.5 mg per 5–8 ounces
Brewed teas	20–110 mg per 5–8 ounces
Iced teas	less than 70 mg per 12 ounces
Soft drinks	up to 54 mg per 12 ounces (depending on brand)

Importantly, approximately half of consumed caffeine stays in the body from
3.5 to 7 hours. Therefore, if a patient drinks two cups of coffee, totaling 200 mg,

at 4 P.M., later that evening at 11 P.M. 100 mg may be left in the patient's body where it can produce nervousness and sleep problems (Olin et al., 1998).

Other medication guidelines that may benefit patients include the following:

- Take medication only as prescribed by the doctor; do not hesitate to call the doctor's office or the pharmacist if you have questions about the medications' compatibility with other medications you may be taking.
- Do not take other peoples' medications.
- Do not take any over-the-counter (OTC) or other drugs without consulting with the doctor or pharmacist first. Always read OTC warnings carefully and make yourself fully aware of side effects.
- Do not stop medication when you feel better. Discontinue only upon the doctor's instruction. The reason to stop taking a medication is *not* because the medication is working!
- Use reminders to assist you in remembering to take medication at correct times and in the right amounts. Common problems with obtaining optimal effects of medications are that people: (a) forget to take them, (b) get tired of taking them, and (c) take forgotten doses too close to the next dose.
- Inform the doctor about all side effects and the continuing course of main effects. Ask the doctor which side effects may be temporary, which can be helped, and which are expected, if not pleasant.
- Ask the doctor or pharmacist any questions you have regarding the medication, no matter how trivial they may seem to you or what others tell you who may be taking a similar drug.
- Counselors: Coach clients to work with doctors as partners in wellness and to discuss concerns openly.

PART 2: HOW MEDICATIONS FUNCTION IN THE BODY AND THE BRAIN

PHARMACOKINETICS AND PHARMACODYNAMICS

PHARMACOKINETICS

The term *pharmacokinetics* refers to the study of in vivo (occurring inside the body) drug processes and includes administration and absorption, distribution, metabolism, and excretion of drugs. Pharmacodynamics refers to the study of the processes by which drugs affect the body and the brain, and the behavioral, emotional, and cognitive outcomes of drug action and neurotransmitter interaction. Gaining a basic understanding of kinetic variables in these processes can provide therapists with the knowledge to recognize, for example, when clients's eating and dosing habits may interfere with a drug's intended effects. An understanding of pharmacodynamics can help therapists understand how the brain communicates with itself and with the body, and how psychiatric drugs interact with neurotransmitters to alter their levels, activities, and interactions, and, in turn, alter cognitive and emotional life.

ADMINISTRATION AND ABSORPTION OF MEDICATIONS

Various methods are available for administering drugs (i.e., oral, intramuscular, intravenous, etc.). The rate of a medication's absorption into the bloodstream is regulated by the method of administration, so the choice of method

---

Box 1-1   Dosing Schedules for Administration of Drugs

Abbreviations used in patient charts to represent common intermittent dosing schedules are:

qid (4 times a day)   gd (every day)
tid (3 times a day)   hs (at bedtime)
bid (2 times a day)   am (in the morning)
ac (before meals)   pm (in the evening)
pc (after meals)

With intermittent dosing, drug levels in the blood will fluctuate. Continuous methods of administering drugs avoid shifts in drug levels. A continuous intravenous method of administration prevents fluctuating drug levels in the blood.

---

1. Oral   3. sublingual (tongue)
2. Injections   4. buccal (cheek & gum)

is an important variable in drug therapy. Drugs that are given intermittently are administered according to specific schedules. Box 1-1 lists common intermittent dosing schedules.

ORAL DRUG ADMINISTRATION

Oral drug forms include liquids, tablets, and capsules. Liquid dosage forms have the fastest absorption rate. Tablets are absorbed more slowly. Capsules are often formulated as time-release or sustained-release products and have the advantage of requiring fewer daily doses. A variety of problems may occur with oral drug administration, including stomach and intestinal problems.

Oral administration is the slowest method of absorption, and the onset of a drug's effect is less predictable because drug absorption from the gastrointestinal tract is often erratic. Variables that affect the rate of absorption of a drug are related to the concurrent intake of food and the drug's pH (acidity or basicity) relative to the pH values of the stomach and the intestines. Drugs can exist in two interconvertible forms, a water-soluble or ionized form and a lipid-soluble or less ionized form. A drug's lipid-to-water solubility is primarily determined by the pH of the drug relative to the pH of the body fluid that harbors the drug.

Drugs administered orally undergo a process called *first-pass metabolism,* which occurs immediately after the drug is absorbed from the gastrointestinal tract. The blood carries the drug to the liver, where some of the drug is metabolized and thus rendered inactive or unable to exert its desired effect.

INJECTABLE DRUGS

Three basic methods are used for injecting medication: intravenous, intramuscular, and subcutaneous injections. *Intravenous* (into the vein) injection has the fastest absorption rate. Because of this, it is potentially the most dangerous form for injection of medication. *Intramuscular* (into the muscle) injection provides a means for rapid absorption but is not as fast as intravenous injection (e.g., antibiotics). *Subcutaneous* (under a layer of skin) injection is used when a slower and more constant rate of absorption is recommended (e.g., insulin).

Some injectable antipsychotics, such as *Haldol Decanoate* and *Prolixin Decanoate*, are formulated to prolong the effects of the drug. Effects of both injectable drugs can last three to four weeks. Injectable drugs can be used in patients with schizophrenia who are not compliant in taking oral medication (Olin et al., 1998; Ponterotto, 1985).

OTHER METHODS OF MEDICATION ADMINISTRATION

A variety of other methods are used for administering drugs, including *sublingual* (a tablet placed under the tongue) and *buccal* (drug positioned between cheek and gum). In each of these alternate administration methods, a drug is readily absorbed into the bloodstream because of the highly vascular membranes (high number of blood vessels) in each of these areas.

DISTRIBUTION

Once administered and absorbed in the bloodstream, medications are carried to various body tissues via the circulatory system. Blood capillaries deliver drugs to different areas in the body. For most drugs, capillary pores are large enough to allow free passage for the drugs to exit the blood system and exert their effects.

PROTEIN BINDING

Some drugs bind irreversibly to circulating proteins in the plasma or blood. A drug that becomes protein-bound is usually so large that it is unable to exit the capillary, rendering it inactive in the bloodstream until separation from the protein. Drug protein binding also hinders a drug's metabolism and excretion, thus causing a drug to remain in the body longer, which increases the drug's half-life.

The term **half-life** is used to describe the average time required to eliminate one-half of a drug's dose. Theoretically, about six half-lives are needed to remove almost all drugs. Therefore, if a drug has a half-life of 4 hours, after 24 hours (6 half-lives times 4-hour half-life) nearly all the drug will be excreted. Drugs with short half-lives require a more frequent dosing schedule than drugs with long half-lives. Drugs with longer half-lives may be particularly dangerous in case of overdose because it takes the body longer to eliminate them.

LIPID SOLUBILITY

A drug's passage across various membranes or barriers in the body, such as the stomach, intestines, blood-brain barrier (BBB), and placenta, depends on a drug's lipid (fat) solubility. Drugs with a high lipid solubility cross the BBB easily and remain in the brain tissues longer than water-soluble drugs do. This difference is explained by the fact that lipid-soluble chemicals or drugs are stored in the body's fat tissue. Unlike many categories of medication, psychotropic medications and drugs of abuse can cross the BBB and reach the central nervous system rather easily.

METABOLISM

Most drugs are metabolized or broken down in the body by liver enzymes, which act to transform chemicals or drugs into more water-soluble (or hydrophilic) entities so the drugs can be excreted in the urine. Because of the decline in liver activity among the elderly, it takes them longer to metabolize drugs. Therefore, drug dosages for the geriatric population are usually reduced. Therapists can help their older clients by paying close attention to their medications' effects. Because of slower metabolism in this population, it is easier for older adults to become quickly overmedicated. Risks of overmedicating are also of particular concern among persons with heart, liver, and kidney disease.

EXCRETION

The kidney is the body's main excretory organ. Therefore, a client with kidney problems may accumulate more drugs in the body, thus requiring smaller doses. Less frequently, drugs are eliminated from the body via the lungs, sweat glands, saliva, feces, bile, and breast milk.

SIDE EFFECTS, INTERACTIONS, CONTRAINDICATIONS, AND TOXICITY

MEDICATION SIDE EFFECTS

Other terms used to describe drug side effects are *adverse reactions* and *untoward* or *unwanted effects.* Rather than being selectively carried to a specific or targeted area, drugs are widely distributed throughout the body. Therefore, a drug will bind with any receptor that its chemical structure will allow. This nonselective drug-binding capacity explains the origin of drug side effects. Adverse drug side effects must be monitored, and a drug's benefits should outweigh any detrimental side effects. Generally, as the dosage is increased, symptoms of the disease decrease but side effects increase. Consequently, adjusting the dose usually alleviates the side effects. Physicians try to determine the best drug dose to alleviate disease symptoms with the least number of side effects. Another common method used to decrease or lessen side effects of a drug is to have **drug holidays**, blocks of time when the drug is not administered.

A **drug allergy** is different from side effects of a drug. An allergy involves histamine reaction. Any amount of the drug can elicit an allergic response. Therefore, a dosage reduction will not prevent an allergic reaction and when allergic reactions occur, the medication is discontinued. Allergic reactions can range from mild to severe and are sometimes fatal. Examples of allergic reactions are hives and difficulty breathing.

DRUG INTERACTIONS

Factors that contribute to drug interactions include **protein binding** and **enzyme induction** or **inhibition**.

PROTEIN BINDING.   Two drugs can compete for binding sites on circulating plasma proteins. Initiating therapy with drug B, which has a high affinity for protein binding, can displace drug A, which is already bound to plasma proteins. This type of drug interaction can be dangerous because of the possibility that toxic blood levels of released drug A may result.

ENZYME INDUCTION OR INHIBITION.   One drug can accelerate the metabolism of another drug by inducing or activating liver enzymes that mediate a drug's metabolism. Conversely, inhibition of hepatic (liver) enzymes by one drug can increase the drug level in the blood and, in turn, increase the pharmacological activity of another drug. Among certain populations, such as cancer patients who require frequent pain medication, liver enzymes may increase resulting in more rapid metabolism of a drug and thus the need for a higher dose to achieve the same effect.

CONTRAINDICATIONS

It is important that clients be honest with doctors about medical history and preexisting conditions. For example, certain medications would not be prescribed for clients with any history of seizures.

TOXICITY

A drug or specific drug dosage is said to be toxic when it damages the brain or other vital organs in the body. Some drugs are toxic at low dosages; other drugs require a larger dosage to inflict brain or organ damage. When a drug requires only a small amount to produce its desired effects, this drug is said to have a low therapeutic dose. If this same drug with the low therapeutic dose also has a high toxic dose, the drug is described as having a large or wide **therapeutic window**. Lithium is an example of a drug with a narrow therapeutic window: there is only a small difference between its effective and toxic doses. A therapeutic window is the range of dosages wherein a drug is both safe and effective.

SUMMARY

Referring clients for medical evaluations arouses ambivalent feelings for many counselors, many of whom have biases against psychotropic medications. Today, however, most therapists will find themselves working with a more difficult client population than in years past. Most practices include many clients who are already taking psychotropic medications, or who need to be referred for a medical/psychiatric evaluation. Therapists who do not educate themselves about this important area face increased ethical dilemmas and legal risks. They also unnecessarily narrow their range of effective practice. They potentially inhibit clients from making their best use of an important resource. Therapists need to be able to work collaboratively as part of a formal or informal multidisciplinary team which includes physicians. Therapists who take the time to learn about medications will communicate observations more effectively to physicians, teach clients to communicate with physicians more effectively, and can, with more credibility, educate physicians about the value of therapy concurrent with medication.

We discussed client symptoms and behaviors that warrant referral for a medical evaluation and included a sample referral letter to a physician. Therapists are increasingly expected to have a broad understanding of clients' experiences with medications, to help clients comply with medical advice, and to help educate clients about medication use and misuse. Also, managed care, insurance reimbursement, and political agendas impact psychotherapy practice. Most critically, therapists face the challenge of how to provide adequate services in the face of shrinking resources. Finally, educating clients about what behaviors enhance the therapeutic benefits of medications will contribute to increased client stability, quality of life, decreased relapse frequency, and need for hospitalization.

PHARMACODYNAMICS AND THE NEUROLOGICAL BASIS OF MENTAL DISORDERS

The human nervous system is a composite of numerous intricate and interactive subsystems that collaborate in the production of human behaviors: thinking, acting, and feeling. Interaction within and between these subsystems is determined by the secretion of chemical messengers, neurotransmitters. Faulty neurological function, often represented by defects in neurotransmitter activity or structural difficulties, may result in emotional or mental disorders that are not fully comprehensible to counselors without an introductory knowledge of neuropharmacology and pharmacopsychology. Further, clients often want and need to understand the broad outlines of what their medications accomplish and why they experience neurological (main) effects and side effects. If counselors do not have a clear understanding of the fundamentals of neurotransmission themselves, they cannot instruct their clients. Thus, demystification for both counselors and clients is the primary focus of this chapter. We hope this discussion will pique your interest in this area and serve as a basis to move ahead into reading or course work emphasizing what has become an explosion of information in neuropsychology and pharmacopsychology. Those who want a more detailed presentation of these topics should consult *A Primer of Drug Action* (Julien, 1998) and progress to *The Biochemical Basis of Neuropharmacology* (Cooper, Bloom, & Roth, 1991); both are well updated and accessible by independent study.

REGULATING EMOTION

Neurotransmission does not merely exercise strategic control over the processes of thinking, feeling, behaving, and the integration of the three; from our perspective it *is* these processes. They are inseparably bound. Each is the transitional end point of a complex neural process elaborated through 30 million years of primate evolution resulting in the ability of Homo sapiens to comprehend themselves and their world. Our design ensures that the brain is not static but can adapt (not always positively) its internal operations to utilize new and novel substances. Thus, the brain is less like a computer than it is like a vast, self-reflective chemistry set, parts of which are dedicated to routine maintenance operations and parts of which are dedicated to novel applications, depending on whether stimuli are from inside or outside the system. When the chemistry set under-, over-, or wrongly produces necessary constituents for neural activity, the system can be adjusted roughly through use of modern medicines that mimic or imitate properties of neurotransmitters. However, it must be emphasized that the adjustment is approximate and that side effects can restrict and negate even the positive aspects of the drug for many individuals. Given the dramatic increase in research on neuroactive drugs, it is clear that future psychiatric medications will allow neurotransmission to be much more finely tuned than we find possible today.

Neurotransmitters (NTs), the primary chemical messengers in the brain, interact with one another and with neuromodulators and hormones to provide the two most important aspects of neural activity. The first is arousal, involving regulation of activity and rest. The second is orientation to time, place, and person, which are the fundamental aspects of consciousness. Arousal and orientation are controlled through the interplay of neurotransmitters, sometimes called **neuromodulators (NM)**, that often work in opponent process to one another and in combination with regulatory neuropeptides (long chains of amino acids). **Opponent process** implies that inhibitory and excitatory neurotransmitters, supported by peptide regulation, are in dynamic equilibrium within many systems of the brain. In a **well-regulated system**, when excitatory activity rises, inhibitory or modulatory activity also rises so that excitation does not spiral out of control. An example of poorly regulated firing of **neurons** occurs in epilepsy, where overfiring may result in seizures.

Further, there is a division of labor within the principal neurotransmitters such that

- some appear more devoted to excitatory processes (norepinephrine)
- some are more devoted to inhibition (gamma-aminobutyric acid, which can produce a calming effect)
- many (possibly most) are either excitatory or inhibitory depending on where they are found in the brain
- some appear to be more regulatory in their effects on specific brain subsystems

Dopamine and serotonin, for example, appear to up- or down-regulate the sensitivity of receptors to norepinephrine while at the same time performing more independent excitatory, inhibitory, or orientation functions within closely related neural systems (Cooper et al., 1991).

The **biological amine hypothesis of depression,** which is well supported by research (Julien, 1996; and which we discuss at length in Chapter 2), indicates that depression can be roughly equated with a lack of excitatory neurotransmitters (or an inability to process them effectively) or an overabundance of neurotransmitters whose function is to inhibit neurotransmission. For example, after a period of prolonged excitement or activity, many of us experience a low point or depression that comes from exhaustion of excitatory neurotransmitters available in the **neural net** (the nervous systems). Exhaustion of excitatory NTs from chronic anxiety or worry or lengthy mental activity can result in chronic depression that usually lifts once the work–rest routine is in better equilibrium. However, individuals whose brains continue to produce insufficient levels of excitatory neurotransmitters, or who are on medications that restrict that development, or whose mental life has profoundly fatigued the system may become so chronically or profoundly depressed that they need medication. These latter forms of depression and accompanying depressed physical states are often treated with drugs that either mimic or raise the available levels of excitatory neurotransmitters within the brain.

Chronically high levels of excitement or mania and anxiety are treated with drugs (BuSpar or Xanax, for example) that either lower the level of excitatory neurotransmitters or raise the levels or enhance the system's sensitivity to inhibitory neurotransmitters. The efficacy of this treatment strategy is further demonstrated by the fact that illegal or unwise use of drugs that inhibit the availability or activity of excitatory neurotransmitters (alcohol and other sedative hypnotics, for example) typically cause depression.

Similarly, although regulatory neurotransmitter functioning is intimately bound together with all the other neurotransmitters and neuromodulators, an

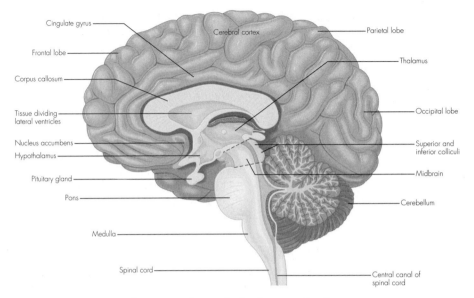

Figure 1-1 A sagittal section through the human brain. *Source:* After Nieuwenhuys, Voogd, & vanHuijzen, 1988; Kalat, 1998.

excess of the (generally excitatory) NT dopamine or oversensitivity to dopamine is known to cause symptoms of psychosis, including disorganization of thought and behavior and, often, paranoia. Conversely, a deficiency of dopamine in the brain has been implicated in overly organized, stereotypic behaviors (continual hand washing, for example) and autism.

Neurotransmitters and neuromodulators activate and orient multiple areas of the brain, the limbic system and the hypothalamus for example, areas of the brain whose duties include regulation of our emotional lives. To provide background for a more complete understanding the physiological basis of emotions, a brief sketch of the nervous system is the focus of Appendix A at the end of the book. For a sketch of the brain, see Figure 1-1.

Figure 1-2 The components of a vertebrate motor neuron. The cell body of a motor neuron is located in the spinal cord. The various parts are not drawn to scale: in particular, a real axon is much longer in proportion to the size of the soma. *Source:* Kalat, 1998.

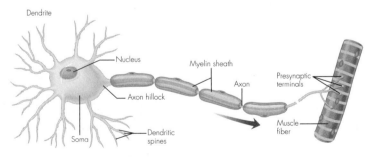

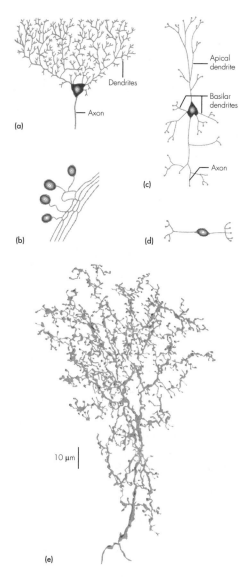

Figure 1-3   The diverse shape of neurons. (a) Purkinje cell, a cell type found only in the cerebellar sensory neurons from skin to spinal cord; (b) sensory neurons from skin to spinal cord; (c) pyramidal cell of the motor area of the cerebral cortex; (d) bipolar cell of the eye; (e) Kenyon cell, from a honey bee.

NEURONS

Neurons are highly specialized nerve cells that conduct impulses throughout the brain and the body (see Figures 1-2 and 1-3). Knowing the characteristics of a neuron can assist in the understanding of the way drugs exert their effects. Like all animal cells, neurons have the following features:

[*] *Cell membrane*: the outer covering of a neuron composed of a double layer of <u>lipid</u> (fatlike) molecules. Many protein molecules floating inside the lipid membrane have special functions, such as detecting specific substances and relaying information about these substances.

[•] *Nucleus*: contains chromosomes (genetic material), which are long strands of DNA, and ribosomes, which function in protein synthesis. Proteins are important not only because they provide cell structure but also because they serve as **enzymes**. Enzymes <u>act as catalysts for chemical</u> <u>reactions in both the synthesis and degradation of molecules.</u> Specific enzymes catalyze specific processes. Some medications act by altering a cell's enzyme activity.

[•] *Cytoplasm*: a jellylike substance that occupies space inside the neuron.

Many other components are also found in a neuron. However, only the neural components important for understanding pharmacology are mentioned here.

Neurons exist in many shapes and varieties. The special purpose of a neuron determines its shape. Most neurons have four structures or regions:

- **Soma:** the cell body of the neuron in which the nucleus and other vital components of the neuron reside.
- **Dendrite:** the branching area of nerve cells. This dividing structure is similar to the branching of a tree. Dendrites and areas on the soma (and sometimes axons as well) contain **receptors**, which are molecules that receive and react to messages from other neurons. Nerve cell receptor sites are often the targeted location for a drug's action. The point where two neurons meet and relay information is called a **synapse**. Areas between neurons in which chemicals are transmitted are referred to as the **synaptic gap** or **synaptic cleft**. —
- **Axon:** a long slender tube of the neuron that relays electrical impulses from the soma to the terminal buttons of the neuron. The length of axons varies, ranging from a few millimeters in the brain to a meter in the spinal track. In the CNS (central nervous system), axons belonging to neurons of one region group together and project to other areas of the brain. CNS axon bundles are referred to as *fibers* or *nerve fibers*. Outside the CNS, the term *nerve* is used to describe bundles of axons.
- **Terminal buttons:** small knoblike structures at the end of axon clusters. Axons divide into numerous subaxons, and each of these branches of axons ends with a terminal button. **Vesicles** or small sacs inside terminal buttons contain neurotransmitters that are released after a relayed impulse reaches the end of the axon.

GLIAL CELLS

Glial cells, also referred to as *neuroglia*, are support cells of the nervous system. Functions of glial cells include, for example:

holding the CNS together (like glue). Glial cells form a matrix to keep neurons in place.

protecting neurons. Glial cells physically and chemically buffer neurons. CNS neurons can be destroyed by head injury, infection, stroke, or other insults. When a neuron dies, it cannot be replaced; therefore the protective assistance of glial cells is important.

cleaning up particles of dead cells.

insulating neurons from other neurons. By surrounding and isolating synapses, glial cells aid in preventing neural messages from being scrambled.

producing **myelin sheaths**. A myelin sheath (see Figure 1-2) is a series of segments forming a tube around the axon of a neuron. Myelin is composed of 80% lipid (fat) and 20% protein.

In the peripheral nervous system (PNS), Schwann cells produce myelin to support and protect peripheral nerve cells. If a PNS axon is damaged, Schwann cells grow a protective tube to help direct new sprouts of the axon to muscles and sense organs. Unfortunately, glial cells in the central nervous system (CNS) cannot perform the same task to repair damaged CNS neurons. CNS glial cells also produce scar tissue that blocks reconnection of new sprouts, a problem to be overcome as we try to regenerate nerves to reconnect different parts of the body after injury.

BLOOD-BRAIN BARRIER

Years ago, a psychologist found that a trypan dye injected into an animal's bloodstream would tint all blood tissues except the brain and spinal cord. Yet, if the dye were injected into the brain's ventricles, the blue dye would spread throughout the CNS. This discovery led to a greater understanding of the structures and the functioning of the CNS.

The **blood-brain barrier (BBB)** is responsible for restricting the dye from dispersing from the blood into the brain tissues. This barrier between the circulating blood in the brain and the fluid that surrounds the brain tissue is composed of astrocytes, a type of glial cell that forms the physical basis of the BBB by encapsulating the capillaries in the brain. Understanding the characteristics of the BBB is of vital importance in the field of pharmacology because the BBB is selectively permeable; that is, some substances (or drugs) gain entry to the CNS easily and others do not. Substances essential to the survival of neurons easily cross the BBB because of an active transport process. **Lipophilic molecules,** those that dissolve readily in fats (for example, those with low ionization), move effortlessly through the BBB. Alcohol is a lipophilic substance that not only can permeate the brain but also permeates the cells and nuclei of cells in the brain, where it acts as a toxin. Thus, alcohol's easy access into neurons explains its rapid effects on one's cognitive and emotional functioning.

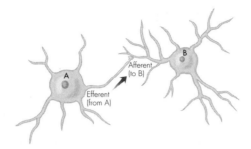

Figure 1-4   Cell structure and axons. It all depends on the point of view. An axon from A to B is an *efferent* axon from A; it is an *afferent* axon to B—just as a train from Washington to New York is *exiting* Washington and *approaching* New York. *Source:* Kalat, 1998.

COMMUNICATION BETWEEN NEURONS

As we have stated in other parts of this chapter, human behavior (thinking, feeling, perceiving, and acting) is the direct result of interaction between nerve cells. Neurons, of which there are approximately 20 billion in the brain, communicate with other neurons by way of chemicals called *neurotransmitters*. In the synaptic cleft (a gap of approximately one 10,000th of an inch; see Figures 1-4 and 1-5), chemical neurotransmitters are released, travel to receptors, and generally produce either an excitatory or inhibitory message on the receiving neuron. An excitatory message increases the likelihood that an impulse will be

Figure 1-3   Some of the major events in transmission at a synapse. *Source:* Kalat, 1998.

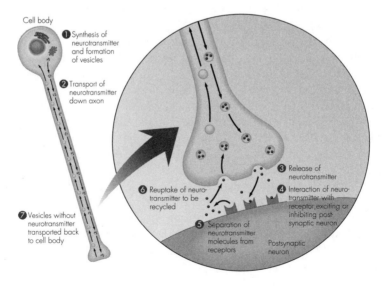

relayed, and an inhibitory message decreases the possibility that the impulse will be transmitted. All neurons can receive both excitatory and inhibitory impulses simultaneously. Therefore, whether a neuron relays a message down its axon depends on the relative activity (number) of the excitatory and inhibitory messages it receives.

The relationship of a neuron to its surrounding tissues is very complex. One neuron can have tens of thousands of synapses on its membrane, allowing a neuron to be the recipient of information from many different neurons. This influx of information, from as many as 50,000 dendrites from various sources into one neuron, is called **convergence**.

Generally, a neuron has only one axon; however, each axon branches into as many as 10,000 terminal buttons. Axonal branching is most profuse in the brain and most elaborate there in the memory systems. When an impulse is transmitted down the axon, it is conveyed to all axial branches. This branching allows a neuron to simultaneously send information to many other neurons, creating **divergence of information**.

ELECTRICAL PROPERTIES OF A NEURON.   Often the electrical properties of a neuron relate to a drug's action. A neuron's electrical charge is attributed to the difference in intracellular (within the neuron) and extracellular (outside the neuron) ion concentrations. **Ions** are small electrically charged molecules. Extracellular fluid is rich in sodium ions (chemically symbolized as $Na+$) and chloride ions ($Cl-$) and the intracellular fluid is rich in potassium ($K+$) and protein ions ($A-$). In a neuron's unexcited state, the average electrical difference between the intracellular and extracellular fluid is 70 millivolts (mV). The term *resting potential* is used to describe a neuron's unexcited state. The electrical charge when a neuron is at its resting potential is -70 mV.

ION EXCHANGE.   Recall that a neuron's membrane is a double layer of lipid molecules, called a *fluid mosaic*, which helps maintain the intracellular–extracellular ion concentration gradient. Molecules inside the neural membrane act as ion pumps or ion channels. When activated, these ion channels allow passage of specific ions (like neurotransmitters or drugs) across a membrane.

Several types of ion channels, differing in method of activation, exist in the neural membrane. The *voltage-dependent ion channel* is activated by changes in the membrane's electrical potential. The *neurotransmitter-dependent ion channel* is activated when neurotransmitters stimulate receptors that directly or indirectly open specific ion gates. Four types of neurotransmitter-dependent ion channels are known. Each causes either an inhibitory or excitatory response. They are:

- sodium (excitatory)
- chloride (inhibitory)
- potassium (excitatory) and
- calcium (excitatory)

neurotransmitter-dependent ion channels

Activation of a specific ion channel is determined by both the particular neurotransmitter and the specific postsynaptic receptor that signals the ion channel to open (Carlson, 1991; Cooper et al., 1991).

CHANGE IN RESTING POTENTIAL. A neurotransmitter causes a receiving neuron's electrical charge to become either *more negative*, a process called *hyperpolarization*, which produces an inhibitory effect by stabilizing the neural membrane, or *more positive*, a process called *depolarization*, which produces an excitatory effect. Hyperpolarizations are also called *inhibitory postsynaptic potentials* (IPSPs). Depolarizations are also referred to as *excitatory postsynaptic potentials* (EPSPs).

[handwritten: Depolarization = excitatory (DE)]
[handwritten: Hyper polarization = inhibitory (HI)]

COMMUNICATION WITHIN A NEURON

The dendrite is the part of the neuron that branches off toward other cells and receives messages from them. At the dendrite, an activated neurotransmitter-dependent ion channel facilitates a change in intracellular ion concentration. Alterations in the intracellular ion concentration produce either the excitatory (EPSP) or the inhibitory effect (IPSP). The magnitude of the neuron's electrical change is proportional to the degree of stimulation on the neurotransmitter-dependent ion channel. Thus, the more NTs stimulate a postsynaptic dendrite, the greater the likelihood of producing an electrical change.

All EPSPs and IPSPs originating at the dendrites are averaged with all IPSPs or EPSPs generated from synapses directly on the soma or cell body. If a neuron's excitation synapses exert more influence than its inhibitory synapses, an **action potential (AP)** will be initiated at the axon hillock, the point where the neuron's axon connects to its soma. An AP is produced when a neuron's resting potential becomes less negative. The change in the resting potential has to reach a specific level or threshold before generating an AP.

All APs are the same size, yet not all behavioral responses are equal in magnitude. Stronger environmental stimuli produce a higher rate of firing of APs. For example, a bright light or loud sound may cause many APs to fire in a short time period, whereas a weak light or sound may stimulate fewer APs in the same time frame. The higher the firing rate of APs, the stronger the behavioral response will be (Carlson, 1991).

The AP is transmitted toward the axon's terminal buttons. Once it is at the axon's terminal button (or nerve end), the AP causes calcium ion channels in the neural membrane to open, allowing an influx of calcium ions ($Ca++$) to the neuron's terminal button. This influx of calcium ions causes vesicles or small reservoirs filled with neurotransmitters to merge with the membrane and release the neurotransmitters into the synaptic cleft. This process of releasing neurotransmitters is called **exocytosis.**

In the synapse, neurotransmitters diffuse across the extracellular fluid and attach to postsynaptic receptors located on the adjacent neuron's soma or dendrite. At the postsynaptic dendrite or soma, neurotransmitters activate special molecules called *receptors*. Activating a receptor directly or indirectly opens ion channels in the postsynaptic neural membrane, which calls for either excitation or inhibition. Recall that the passage of ions across a neural membrane will cause either hyperpolarization (inhibitory message) or depolarization (excitatory message).

RECEPTOR ACTIVATION.   All neurotransmitters fit into their respective receptors in a way similar to a key in a lock. There are two basic ways a neurotransmitter can open an ion channel. One way is through an acetylcholine receptor. When two acetylcholine (ACh) molecules occupy the two ACh sites on a single receptor, a sodium ion pump is opened, allowing an influx of sodium ions, which produces depolarization (and, therefore, excitation).

The second way an NT can open an ion channel is less direct and more complicated. A neurotransmitter (norepinephrine, for example) can attach to a receptor site, indirectly activating the production of cyclic adenosine monophosphate (cyclic AMP). Cyclic AMP, acting as a second messenger, activates enzymes (molecules that weaken or break down other substances) called *protein kinases*. In turn, protein kinases facilitate a change in the physical shape of proteins that control the opening of an ion channel. The alteration in the physical shape of the protein permits the opening, allowing an influx of ions into the postsynaptic neuron. This ion influx can cause either depolarization or hyperpolarization.

TERMINATION OF ACTIVITY IN THE SYNAPSE.   Postsynaptic potentials are brief. The neurotransmitter's work in the synaptic cleft occurs in a very short period of time, as quickly as one 10,000ths of a second. Two mechanisms halt the action of neurotransmitters in the synapse; they are reuptake and enzymatic deactivation.

Reuptake is a process of extremely rapid removal of the neurotransmitter from the synaptic cleft by the presynaptic neuron's terminal button. Many drugs exert their desired therapeutic effect by influencing this reuptake process. **Enzymatic deactivation** is a degradation process of the neurotransmitter by an enzyme. For example, acetylcholine is destroyed by the enzyme acetylcholinesterase. And catecholamines are broken down for reuptake into the terminal vesicles by the enzymes monoamine oxidase (MAO) and catechol O-methyltransferase (COMT). (Note that enzymes usually end in the suffix *-ase*.)

CHARACTERISTICS OF NEUROTRANSMITTERS

Neurotransmitters and neuromodulators are chemicals that facilitate communication between neurons. NTs differ from NMs in that NMs are released from vesicles in greater quantities than NTs and can travel to other synapses in the brain. NTs usually act in the synapse where they are released.

In 1904, adrenalin (epinephrine) was the first NT to be described in the literature. Today, much information has been accumulated about NTs; however, many unknowns still exist. For example, researchers are not certain whether one neuron produces and releases several different NTs, although it is thought that each neuron produces a primary NT. Variants of that primary NT can, however, lock onto subsets of receptors, and a variety of neuroactive peptides (or NMs in some cases) can interact to condition the interaction of release and binding on the postsynaptic receptor. Scientists continue to identify new endogenous NTs and neuroactive peptides. Some NTs seem to be exclusively excitatory or inhibitory (the amino acid transmitter glycine, for example). Yet other NTs are capable of both inhibition and excitation (dopamine, for example), depending on the nature of the postsynaptic receptor an NT activates.

⦁ Neurotransmitters are commonly classified into four groups:

1. **Catecholamines**, so named because these NTs are derived from a compound called *catechol* and have an amine group. NTs included in this group are dopamine (DA), norepinephrine (NE), and epinephrine (Epi).
2. **Monoamines**, a more inclusive grouping system. The only criterion for membership in this class of NTs is belonging to a single amine group. All the catecholamines are also members of the monamine class, which consists of dopamine, norepinephrine, epinephrine, and serotonin or 5-hydroxytryptamine (5-HT).
3. **Amino acids**, building blocks for proteins. Amino acids also act as neurotransmitters in the CNS. Important amino acids include: gama-aminobutyric acid (GABA), glycine, and glutamic acid (glutamate).
4. **Neuropeptides**, chains of amino acids. Included in this group are endorphins and substance P.

✠Major Neurotransmitters✠

Acetylcholine (ACh) is neither a catecholamine nor a monoamine. ACh has major roles in both the PNS and the CNS. In the PNS, ACh is found at synapses where axons meet skeletal muscles. At this location, ACh causes excitation leading to muscle contraction. ACh is also widely distributed in the brain. Organic diseases in which ACh is thought to play an important role are Parkinson's disease, Alzheimer's disease, and myasthenia gravis.

Parkinson's disease, a movement disorder, is thought to result from an imbalance of DA and ACh in the basal ganglia of the brain. Dopaminergic neurons (cells that produce DA) degenerate in Parkinson's, resulting in ACh exerting a greater influence than DA. Sometimes, Parkinson's disease is treated with anticholinergic agents (drugs that decrease the action of ACh).

On the other hand, myasthenia gravis, a progressive disease of muscular weakness and fatigability, results from inadequate action of ACh. Myasthenia gravis is treated with drugs called *cholinesterase inhibitors*. Cholinesterase inhibitors suppress the action of the enzyme that breaks down ACh in synapses, thus prolonging the effects of ACh. Cholinesterase inhibitors are often used commercially as insecticides (which can have serious nervous system health consequences for humans who interact with them) and have been and are still employed on humans as lethal nerve gases.

Alzheimer's disease, a progressive disease that results in severe dementia and eventual death, has been associated with a deficiency in brain ACh. Memory deficits noted in Alzheimer's are thought to result, at least partially, from lower ACh levels in the hippocampus (Gossel & Wuest, 1992).

ACh is not only important for proper memory functioning but also plays a role in learning, behavioral arousal, attention, mood, and rapid eye movement (REM) activity that occurs during sleep. Drugs that mimic ACh or potentiate ACh effects facilitate REM sleep.

Epinephrine (Epi) is produced by the adrenal gland, a small endocrine gland located above the kidney. Epi exerts most of its effects in the PNS, where it functions to maintain heart rate and blood pressure. Epi is active in the brain but is not as important in neurotransmission as norepinephrine. **Adrenalin** is another term used for Epi.

Norepinephrine (NE) is primarily an excitatory NT. In the CNS, cell bodies of neurons that produce NE are located in the brain stem, with their axons projecting into the limbic system (a group of brain structures involved in emotions) and into the frontal lobes. NE is also involved in maintaining wakefulness and alertness. In the PNS, NE is active in "fight or flight" responses. When released in the spinal cord, NE exerts an analgesic effect by slowing the release of an NT called **substance P**, which activates pain reception.

Dopamine (DA) can produce both excitatory and inhibitory effects in the CNS. DA is thought to be involved in movement, learning, and attention. As described earlier, Parkinson's disease is caused by a deficiency of DA. One treatment for Parkinson's disease is to administer the drug L-dopa, a precursor to DA. L-dopa can cross the BBB, whereas DA cannot. Once in the brain, some of the L-dopa is converted to DA. Overactivity of DA or oversensitivity of DA receptors is linked with symptoms of schizophrenia. Parkinson's patients treated with L-dopa occasionally have side effects similar to symptoms of schizophrenia. And, in the same vein, side effects of phenothiazine drugs (which deplete DA and are, therefore, used in treatment of schizophrenia) often produce the involuntary movements characteristic of Parkinson's disease. Two types of DA receptors have been isolated, called D1 and D2. Amphetamine and cocaine, two frequently abused drugs, activate DA receptors; this activation of DA receptors produces stimulating and reinforcing properties (excitation) and also helps account for the schizophrenialike behaviors common to large-scale or long-term use of these drugs.

Serotonin (5-HT) is thought to be involved in the inhibition of activity and behavior. It is active in mood regulation, control of eating, sleep and arousal, and pain regulation. Axons of NE and 5-HT project into almost the same areas of the brain; NE and 5-HT are thought to have opposing actions in these areas. Antidepressant drugs, particularly the heterocyclics like fluoxetine (Prozac) and sertraline (Zoloft), work principally by blocking the reuptake of 5-HT (Beasley, Masica, & Potvin, 1992; Reimherr et al., 1990; Stahl, 1992).

Gamma-aminobutyric acid (GABA) is an amino acid that functions as an inhibitory NT by making the brain more stable and preventing overexcitation of neurons. Several sedating drugs, such as the benzodiazepines and barbiturates, are active at GABA receptor site complexes.

Glutamate is an excitatory amino acid NT that lowers the threshold for neural excitation. It is often in oriental food in the form of monosodium gluta- MSG mate. After ingesting large quantities of glutamate, individuals sensitive to glutamate may experience dizziness and other transient but mild neurological symptoms.

Glycine is another amino acid. Glycine has inhibitory effects in the spinal cord, where it is highly concentrated. The poison strychnine blocks glycine, thus preventing glycine's inhibitory action, resulting in continual seizures. If an antidote for this poison is not administered quickly, death usually results (Klaassen, 1993).

Neuropeptides, or neuromodulators, unlike amino acid and monoamine NTs that come from dietary sources, are produced within cells in ribosomes where their synthesis is directed by messenger RNA (mRNA). Neuropeptides are composed of chains of amino acids and are intermediate between amino acids and proteins in size.

Figure 1-6   Synapses responsible for pain and its inhibition. The pain afferent neuron releases substance P as its neurotransmitter. Another neuron releases enkephalin at presynaptic synapses; the enkephalin inhibits the release of substance P and therefore alleviates pain. *Source:* Kalat, 1998.

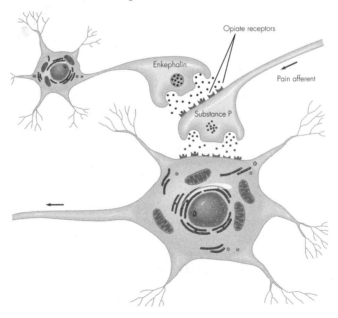

Endorphins or **opioid peptides** are internally manufactured neuropeptides that, like morphine (after which they are named), can produce analgesia, affect the perception of pain, induce respiratory depression, cause sedation, and alter affective behavior and feelings of well-being. **Enkephalins** and **dynorphins** are other terms used to refer to subgroups of these neuromodulators (See Figure 1-6). As there are different varieties of endorphins, various types of CNS endorphin receptors exist. Opioid NMs are very specific molecules, meaning that only specific NMs can stimulate certain opioid receptors. The chemical structure of the opioid NM will determine which receptor it can activate.

PHARMACOLOGY IN THE NEURON

Drugs can alter behavior by interrupting or altering any one of the many processes that occur in neural communication. A drug that increases the availability or mimics the action of an endogenous NT is called an **agonist**. Conversely, a drug that decreases the availability or action of an NT is called an **antagonist**. Agonist drug actions include

- being a precursor for an NT, resulting in an increase in NT synthesis increasing release of NTs from terminal buttons
- acting like endogenous NTs and stimulating postsynaptic receptors
- blocking reuptake by presynaptic neurons, allowing NTs to remain in synapse longer and
- immobilizing enzymes that break down NTs in synapse, thus increasing the number of NTs in the synapse available for action (Carlson, 1991)

Antagonist drug actions include

- decreasing the production of an NT by blocking the enzyme required for its synthesis
- blocking storage of NTs in vesicles
- preventing release of NTs (sometimes substance P) from terminal buttons (see Figure 1-6)
- binding postsynaptic receptors without stimulating them, hindering NT activity and
- stimulating receptors on presynaptic neurons, called *autoreceptors*, which tell neurons not to release NTs (Carlson, 1991)

CONCLUSION

We hope this outline of the fundamentals of neurotransmission will enhance your understanding of the discussions presented in the chapters that follow. In reading those chapters, bear in mind that as we achieve a deeper understanding of neurophysiology, we increase our knowledge of the psychiatric problems that accompany faulty neurotransmission.

CHAPTER 1 REVIEW QUESTIONS

1. Define *pharmacopsychology*.
2. What are the problems therapists face in referring people for evaluation for psychiatric medication?
3. What are the situations that warrant referral to a psychiatrist? Under what conditions should people be referred for medication or inpatient treatment?
4. What do we mean when we say that a psychiatric medication is not a magic bullet?
5. In what domains are therapists most likely to impact clients' compliance with psychiatric medications?
6. List six medication guidelines that may benefit patients.
7. Define *pharmacokinetics*.
8. Define drug *half-life*.
9. Describe the differences between drug side effects and adverse drug reactions, including allergic reactions.
10. Describe two factors that contribute to drug interactions.
11. What is the relationship between neurotransmitters and the regulation of emotions?
12. Name the basic constituents of the neuron and explain their roles in communication between neurons.
13. How is termination of activity in the synapse accomplished?
14. Name six important neurotransmitters and describe how they function.
15. Describe agonist and antagonist actions in the synapse.

WEB RESOURCES FOR PROFESSIONALS

In your Internet browser, either Netscape or Internet Explorer, there is a blank space available where you can type the following URL addresses. URL addresses are universal resource locations that start with the letters "http://" and show you a page of information on the Internet. Type any of the following URL addresses into that space and press return in order to go to that page. A variety of access buttons (highlighted words that you may point to and click on) are available for further information.

Please note that because of the continuously changing sites, we cannot guarantee that pages will remain at these location addresses. If pages are incomplete, use the address without the last part of the extension (instead of using http://www.mentalhealth.com/fr20.html, use only http://www.mentalhealth.com).

A. http://www.mentalhealth.com/fr20.html

What information does this URL address provide?

This page lists descriptions, diagnoses, and treatment and research findings on 52 of the most common mental disorders. (Examples include depression and bipolar disorder). The 67 most common psychiatric drugs (for example, Imipramine and Prozac) including indications, warnings, adverse affects, and dosage are provided.

How can this page be used?

The left side of the screen contains a list of the most common mental disorders. To select a disorder, click on its name.

Information on each disorder includes the following:

American description	Research on diagnosis, treatment, and cause
European description	Information booklets
Treatment information	Magazine articles

The bottom of the screen contains a list of topics. To select topics about medication, diagnosis, or treatment of various disorders, click on its name. Information on medication includes the following:

Pharmacology	Indications
Contraindications	Warnings
Precautions	Adverse Effects

B. http://pharminfo.com/

C. http://www.cmhc.com/guide/pro22.htm

D. http://uhs.bsd.uchicago.edu/~bhsiung/tips/tips.html

Commands to: majordomo@psycom.net Subscribe: subscribe psycho-pharm
Unsubscribe: unsubscribe psycho-pharm List: psycho-pharm@psycom. net

2

DEPRESSION AND ANTIDEPRESSANTS

BIPOLAR DISORDERS AND LITHIUM

This chapter provides an introduction to the underlying somatic and emotional causes of depression and discusses the relationship between its etiology and its treatment. We will pay special attention to the issues of why, when, and how counselors should refer clients to a physician for evaluation concerning antidepressant medication. Finally, we will discuss what is known of the etiology of bipolar disorder (also called *manic-depression*), the psychiatric drugs used in its treatment, and the drug-compliance problems that often arise.

DEPRESSION

Depression is the most common psychiatric disorder in adults after anxieties. Depression, however, is a more life-threatening emotional illness and accounts for approximately 75% of psychiatric hospitalizations; 20% of women and 10% of men experience at least one major depressive episode in their lives (Fuller & Underwood, 1989). The potential danger of depression is illustrated by the fact that severely depressed patients are at high risk for suicide. Approximately 80% of suicidal individuals have depressive illnesses.

In addition to suicide risks associated with depression, depressive illnesses may be as physically and mentally disabling as a severe chronic medical illness. Depressed employees in the work force are less productive, have more accidents, and file more disability claims. Collectively, mood disorders are the most costly mental illness (Hall & Wise, 1995).

Depression is considered a mood illness, whereas schizophrenia is a disease primarily interfering with perception and thought processes. Schizophrenia does, however, produce severe secondary depressive episodes that are often as disabling as the thought disorder itself. These secondary depressive episodes produce active psychoses in 10 to 15% of depressed clients with schizophrenia (Jonas & Schaumburg, 1991).

DIAGNOSIS

An estimated 50–60% of individuals with significant depression are not properly diagnosed. Symptoms of depression are often misattributed to other health problems and can go undiagnosed for many years or a lifetime (Hall & Wise, 1995). The *Diagnostic and Statistical Manual of Mental Disorders, Fourth Edition* (DSM-IV) (American Psychiatric Association, 1994) describes the criteria for a diagnosis of depression. A feeling of depressed mood or loss of pleasure in almost all activities that lasts for at least two weeks is the essential feature of a major unipolar depressive episode.

Depressed clients are often unable to cope and are immobilized without understanding why. They often feel guilty for their lack of self-efficacy and self-esteem and are shamed by their condition. This sense of shame further restricts their range of social interactions, which further reinforces their view of themselves as inadequate.

Although the average age of onset for depression is late 20s, it may occur much earlier (APA, 1994). Depression in children, as in the elderly, is less well researched (Waterman & Ryan, 1993) and is often misdiagnosed, underreported, and undertreated. The link between many childhood behavioral disorders (attention-deficit hyperactivity disorder, for example) and depression is only now being explored (Gadow, 1992; Klein, 1987). For an update on attention-deficit hyperactivity disorders (ADHD), see Pelham (1993). Further, exploration of the relationship between chronic pain, chronic fatigue, **fibromyalgia**, and depression among adults has also been neglected until very recently. These conditions are clearly interconnected. Further, Cassem (1995) suggests that utilization of medical outpatient facilities could be greatly reduced by more accurate detection of depressive disorders.

[handwritten margin note: pain in soft fibrous tissues of body]

UNIPOLAR DEPRESSION SUBTYPES

Unipolar depression encompasses a large group of heterogenous conditions that include major depression, dysthymia, and minor depression. A broad distinction can be made among the many depression classification systems. The depression subtypes *biological, endogenous,* and *primary* can be contrasted with another cluster of depression types that include *reactive, situational, exogenous,* and *secondary* (Lawson & Copperrider, 1988). As implied by the names, the etiology or precipitating factors are somewhat different between the two broad groupings. The former cluster is suspected to occur because of a spontaneous biochemical imbalance in the brain and is thought to have a genetic basis, even though environmental triggers, such as stress, may exist. This genetic predisposition plus its triggering mechanism is often referred to as a *stress-diathesis model* of depression. The latter cluster of depression types is considered to be a secondary response to external events, such as personal loss, financial problems, health problems, or administration of certain medications. Swonger and Matejski (1991) estimate that 20% of the cases of major depressive episodes are endogenous and 80% are exogenous. Interestingly, the symptoms and recovery rates for situational and nonsituational depressions are comparable, even though the relapse rate and lethality appears higher in endogenous depression (Hammen, 1991).

DYSTHYMIA.   A further important subdivision of unipolar depression is the distinction drawn in DSM-IV between major depression, which is either episodic and acute (or even seasonal), and *dysthymia* or depressive neurosis. **Dysthymia** is a subacute form of depression that is continuous for a minimum of two years (one year in children). Its symptoms are present without breaks of more than two months, and it is chronic. Dysthymia, like major depression, is thought to be both endogenously and exogenously caused. Symptoms of major depression are either not present in dysthymia, not present for long, or are in remission. The client often feels fatigue, low self-esteem, hopelessness, and may have either a poor appetite or overeat. The client may have insomnia or hypersomnia, poor concentration, or difficulty making decisions. Dysthymia is often divided into two groups: primary and secondary. Primary dysthymia is not caused by other DSM-IV Axis I nonmood disorders (for example, schizophrenia or substance abuse) or by Axis III medical disorders. Secondary dysthymia is thought to be caused by a chronic DSM-IV Axis I or Axis III disorder.

Dysthymic individuals found to have a major depressive episode are said to suffer from **double depression** and are high risks for both accident and suicide.

MINOR DEPRESSION.   Minor depression includes dysthymia, cyclothymia, depression not otherwise specified, and adjustment disorder with depressed mood. These conditions are good candidates for antidepressant drug treatment *if psychotherapy has not made a significant difference in the level of depression after three months* (Stewart, Quitkin, & Klein, 1992).

DRUGS THAT PRODUCE DEPRESSION.   Some drugs are known to produce exogenous or secondary types of depression (see Box 2-1). Therapists should pay special attention to all drugs their clients are taking, including over-the-counter (OTC) and abusable drugs that may cause depression or other psychiatric conditions.

ꝑ Box 2-1   Drugs Associated with Exogenous Depression

Sedative–Hypnotic Agents
Alcohol
Benzodiazepines (see Chapter 3)
Barbiturates (see Chapter 3)
Equanil (meprobamate)
Noctec (chloral hydrate)

**Anti-Inflammatory and
Analgesic Agents**
Butazolidin (phenylbutazone)
Indocin (indomethacin)
Opioids or narcotics (see Chapter 5)
Talwin (pentazocine)

Steroids
Corticosteroids
Estrogen withdrawal
Oral contraceptives

Over-the-Counter Drugs
Antihistamines

Miscellaneous Agents
Antineoplastic agents (used for cancers)
Anti-Parkinson drugs (see Chapter 4)
Antipsychotic drugs (see Chapter 4)
Myambutal Ethambutol (used for tuberculosis)

Other Abusable Drugs
Marijuana
Opium derivatives (morphine, codeine)
Phencyclidine (PCP) (anesthetic psychedelic)

**Antihypertensive and
Cardiovascular Drugs**

Trade Name	Generic Name
Aldomet	Methyldopa
Apresoline	Hydralazine
Catapres	Clonidine
Inderal	Propranolol
Ismelin	Guanethidine
Lanoxin	Digoxin
Lopressor	Metoprolol
Minipress	Prazosin
Pronestyl	Procainamide
Serpasil	Reserpine

Sources: Fuller & Underwood, 1989; Olin et al., 1998; Taylor, 1990.

It is also common for depression to occur secondarily to biological disease processes. Numerous illnesses can precipitate a depressive state. A list of the more common medical conditions associated with depression is included in Box 2-2.

ETIOLOGY

Clients often express guilt and shame for their problems during discussions about the causes of their depression and often have a poor conceptual understanding of how depression interacts in a variety of life areas. Education is not

---

Box 2-2   Medical Conditions Associated with Exogenous Depression

Endocrine Disorders
Addison's disease — *no Epi*
Cushing's disease
Diabetes mellitus
Fibromyalgia
Hyperparathyroidism
Hyperthyroidism
Hypothyroidism

Central Nervous System Disorders
Alzheimer's disease
Brain tumors
Huntington's disease
Multiple sclerosis
Parkinson's disease

Cardiovascular Disorders
Cerebralvascular accident (stroke)
Congestive heart failure
Myocardial infarction

Miscellaneous Disorders
Carcinoma (cancer)
Infectious disease
Malnutrition
Mental retardation
Metabolic abnormalities
Pancreatic disease
Pernicious anemia
Rheumatoid arthritis
Systemic lupus erythematosus

Sources: Fuller & Underwood, 1989; Taylor, 1990.

---

only empowering but can decrease the anxiety and associated learned helplessness. Education about the relationship between mental and physical components is particularly helpful. Sleep problems and changes in physical activity and appetite represent major physical aspects of depression. Education should include an evolving understanding of both physical symptoms and the underlining chemical imbalance in the brain that leads to functional difficulties.

Biological theories of depression are supported by the high prevalence of depression in people with diseases involving the nervous system such as epilepsy, multiple sclerosis, and Parkinson's disease. This correlation suggests that basic neuronal changes have occurred (Cassem, 1995).

The biological amine hypothesis of depression states that there is a functional deficit of the neurotransmitters serotonin (5-HT) or norepinephrine (NE) in the brain. This hypothesis is supported by the fact that antidepressants increase levels of NE and 5-HT along with alleviating many of the signs and symptoms of depression. Other evidence offered as support for this hypothesis is that drugs like reserpine, which lower blood pressure, also lower central nervous system levels of NE and 5-HT and produce depression. Further support is provided from research that has shown mania (the behavioral opposite of depression) to result from an overabundance of NE in the synaptic cleft.

However, it is suspected that the biological amine model of depression is too simplistic. The reason for this suspicion is that although the effects of antidepressant medications (AMs) on brain levels of NE and 5-HT are immediate, the reversal of depressive symptoms is delayed two to six weeks after the initiation of antidepressant therapy. A more sophisticated theory would explain the triggering and feedback systems in the brain that may account for the delayed action. It is reasonable to assume that the brain does not simply interpret a rise in arousal produced by excitatory neurotransmitters as an end to depression. Depression is a complex affective syndrome that includes low arousal, changes in the levels of a number of neurotransmitters responsible for both orientation and arousal, and individual interpretation of internal and external states. Further, our experience as therapists indicates that depressed individuals do not necessarily recognize the early movement out of depression, even though we may see clear changes in the client's mood, thinking, and behavior. It is therefore of great importance that we help clients accurately track their therapeutic movement and instill hope.

It is crucial to recognize that many suicides occur during phases when the client feels more capable of action (vegetative, physical symptoms are improving) but feels no less emotionally overwhelmed by the depression (nonvegetative symptoms are not improving). Attention should be focused for a definite period of time during each session on suicide issues and, if necessary, on (control) contracts that include realistic crisis-management steps. Finally, and particularly warranted by continued deterioration of impulse control or substance abuse, orderly steps for inpatient treatment need to be discussed with the client.

TREATMENT OF DEPRESSION

Though depression is the most common mental or emotional problem leading to psychotherapy, most people do not seek treatment (Hammen, 1991). Further, 60% of depressed persons who do seek treatment are misdiagnosed as suffering from other problems (Restak, 1988). Finally, among those who take antidepressant medications (AMs), 30–50% discontinue the drug before treatment effects can take place or are prescribed a dose below the effective treatment dosage (Kimberly et al., 1992).

Depression can impede physical, psychological, and social functioning. The combination of adverse physiological effects and emotional instability frequently leads depressed patients to suicidal ideation. Further, approximately 50% of people with a history of depression among first-degree relatives will have depressive episodes (Restak, 1988).

Accurate assessment and proper treatment of depression, which often requires both psychotherapy and drug interventions, have been shown to restore normal functioning in a majority of clients and also reduce overall medical costs (Hall & Wise, 1995). Therefore, clients should be educated on the benefits of psychotherapy and medication options. Studies comparing the efficacy of drug treatment for depression with psychotherapy have not found significant differences. However, bimodal treatment, which includes both psychotherapy and antidepressant medication, improves the recovery rate for depression over and above either intervention used alone. Emotional coping and social functioning are aided primarily by psychotherapy, while the physiological symptoms are helped by antidepressants. The beneficial effects of exercise and diet on the physiological symptoms of depression should not be underestimated. For cases of severe depression that are unresponsive to drug treatment and psychotherapy, electroconvulsive therapy (ECT) is available.

Generally, ECT is reserved for treatment of patients with severe depression (or severe mania) and a history of failure with drug therapy. ECT is also used with patients who cannot take antidepressants because of medical problems (Ellenor & Dishman, 1996). Sackeim (1997) reports that 70–90% of depressed patients who are treated with ECT show marked improvement shortly after initiation of treatment. When remission of depression is achieved by ECT treatment, special attention must be placed on pharmacological strategies and psychotherapy to prevent relapse. Since many of the patients who receive ECT have been unresponsive to drug treatment, it is recommended that practitioners develop a detailed assessment of the effectiveness of past antidepressant treatments. Unfortunately, relapse rates in the first six months following ECT reach approximately 80%. Maintenance or continued ECT has been effective in many difficult cases, however, and this practice on an outpatient basis is growing (Sackeim, 1997).

Unmedicated episodes of major depression usually last between four and six months (APA, 1994). If a patient has two or more depressive episodes within a relatively short time period and has a history or family history of positive responses to antidepressant agents, then long-term prophylactic AM treatment may be warranted. Prophylactic treatment (treatment that generally lasts longer than one year and is given to forestall a relapse) should not be unsupervised for a variety of reasons: Side effects may, over time, begin to outweigh therapeutic effects of the drug and antidepressant medications are expensive, often costing more than $100 per month, and clients often weigh their therapeutic advantages against their costs. However, newer, less toxic forms of antidepressant medications may soon be available.

REFERRAL CONSIDERATIONS.   Studies have shown that depression relapses occur when antidepressants are discontinued soon after the acute symptoms have been controlled (Hammen, 1991). Relapse is less likely to occur when antidepressant medications are continued at least six months after the acute symptoms have abated (Reimherr et al. 1998). Reimherr also indicates that patients with chronic depression may need antidepressant medication for a year or more. Relapse into a major depressive episode is less likely to occur after medications are discontinued if psychotherapy has been initiated. In their classic study, *The Cognitive Therapy of Depression*, Beck, Rush, Shaw, and Emery (1979) provide a list of characteristics to consider when deciding whether cognitive therapy, antidepressant therapy, or a combination of therapies should be undertaken (see Box 2-3). Although their discussion is directed at cognitive therapy options, other forms of psychotherapy shown to be effective in cases of depression may be generalized.

Box 2-3 ✗Choosing an Appropriate Plan for Therapy

Criteria that would justify administration of cognitive therapy alone
1. Failure to respond to adequate trials of two different AMs
2. Partial response to adequate doses of AMs
3. Failure to respond or only partial response to other psychotherapies
4. Diagnosis of minor affective disorder
5. Variable mood reactive to environmental events
6. Variable mood that correlates with negative cognitions
7. Mild somatic disturbance symptoms (sleep, appetite, weight, or libidinal)
8. Adequate reality testing (that is, no hallucinations or delusions) and adequate span of concentration and memory function
9. Inability to tolerate medication side effects, or evidence that excessive risk is associated with pharmacotherapy

Situations in which cognitive therapy alone is not indicated
1. Evidence of coexisting schizophrenia, organic brain syndrome, alcoholism, narcotic abuse, or mental retardation
2. Patient has medical illness or is taking medication likely to cause depression
3. Obvious memory impairment or poor reality testing (hallucinations, delusions)
4. History of manic episodes (bipolar depression)
5. History of family member who responded to antidepressant medication
6. History of family member with bipolar illness
7. Absence of precipitating or exacerbating environmental stresses
8. Little evidence of cognitive distortions
9. Presence of severe somatic complaints (for example, pain)

Situations in which medication plus cognitive therapy are appropriate
1. Partial or no response to a trial of cognitive therapy alone
2. Partial but incomplete response to adequate pharmacotherapy alone
3. Poor compliance with medication regimen
4. Historical evidence of chronic maladaptive functioning with depressive syndrome on an intermittent basis
5. Presence of severe somatic symptoms and marked cognitive distortions (for example, hopelessness)
6. Impaired memory and concentration and marked psychomotor difficulty
7. Severe depression with suicidal danger
8. History of first-degree relative who responded to antidepressants
9. History of mania in close relative or in patient

Source: From *Cognitive Therapy of Depression* by A. Beck, A. J. Rush, B. F. Shaw, G. Emery, pp. 366–368, The Guilford Press, 1979. Reprinted by permission of Aaron Beck.

TREATMENT CONSIDERATIONS.   Counselors are routinely faced with several converging problems concerning clients and their use of depression medication. First, counselors are expected to understand the client's point of view regarding problems with their antidepressant. Second, counselors are expected to know the conditions under which clients should be referred to a physician for appraisal for antidepressant medication. Third, counselors are expected to help clients with drug compliance. Fourth, counselors are expected to understand and educate the client about the interactions of their medication and alcohol or illicit drugs and issues of dual diagnosis.

MISCONCEPTIONS ABOUT DEPRESSION AND TREATMENT.   To increase compliance and educate the client, counselors need to explore misconceptions about the client's medications, depression, and psychotherapy. Beck et al. (1979) outlined the cognitions contributing to poor adherence to medication prescription (see Box 2-4).

Other misconceptions about antidepressant medications are that once antidepressant medications are begun they cannot be discontinued due to medical reasons, that the side effects are permanent; that the therapist is responsible for the depression management; that psychotherapy makes it possible to cut back (lower the dose) on the amount of AM; that therapy can completely and permanently cure depression; and that depression will change without clients' examining and possibly changing how they think, act, and feel in a wide range of areas.

Because beliefs that sabotage successful therapy are often subtle and deeply held, coming from the family and from society at large, therapists must engage clients in a dialogue about their beliefs concerning their problems and possible solutions. A willingness and ability to confront these issues, of course, lie at the heart of why counselors are successful in treating depression. During active depression, clients' cognitions are often distorted so that education and rational appraisal of the situation is compromised. Clients are likely to selectively attend to accounts of the usefulness or harmfulness of the drugs they are using. They may unreasonably magnify the meaning and importance of side effects, and because their feedback systems are dulled, clients may be unaware of positive changes in their cognitions and overt behaviors. Counselors must, therefore, ask for client reports on their physical, emotional, and cognitive condition during each counseling session and direct the client toward an understanding of the meaning of these conditions to their overall progress. Counselors must work to keep the client aware of the progress being made without rescuing the client.

REFERRAL.   Depressed clients should be referred to a psychiatrist or family practice physician for appraisal for medications (or for possible hospitalization) when any one of these circumstances is present:

1. Client is at a high risk for suicide. Risk factors include patient history and family history of suicide or high-risk behaviors, present crisis, present depression inventories (Beck Depression Inventory, for example), risk demographics (age, sex, and isolation, for example), threats to harm oneself, and having a feasible plan to implement suicidal actions.

Box 2-4 Client Cognitions Contributing to Poor Drug Compliance

Client cognitions about the medication before taking it
1. It's addicting.
2. I am stronger if I don't need medicine.
3. I am weak to need it (a crutch).
4. It won't work for me.
5. If I don't take medication, I'm not crazy.
6. I can't stand side effects.
7. I'll never get off medication once I start.
8. There's nothing I need to do except take medicine.
9. I only need to take medication on "bad days."

Client cognitions about the medication while taking it
1. Since I'm perfectly well (or not any better) after days or weeks, the medicine isn't working.
2. I should feel good right away.
3. The medicine will solve all my problems.
4. The medicine won't solve problems, so how can it help?
5. I can't stand the dizziness (or fuzziness) or other side effects.
6. It makes me into a zombie.

Client cognitions about depression
1. I am not ill (I don't need help).
2. Only weak people get depressed.
3. I deserve to be depressed since I am a burden on everybody.
4. Isn't depression a normal reaction to the bad state of things?
5. Depression is incurable.
6. I am one of the small percentage that does not respond to any treatment.
7. Life isn't worth living, so why should I try to get over my depression?

Source: From *Cognitive Therapy of Depression* by A. Beck, A. J. Rush, B. F. Shaw, G. Emery, p. 372, The Guilford Press, 1979. Reprinted by permission of Aaron Beck.

---

2. Client exhibits intense vegetative signs, including early morning wakening, melancholia, somatic symptoms (weight loss, insomnia, agitation, or psychomotor restlessness, for example).

3. Client is psychotic (for example, client exhibits severe impairment in reality testing as manifested by hallucinations or delusions).

4. Client has a history of alcohol or other drug abuse or dependence.

5. Client has impairments to memory, attention, or signs of muscle weakness or spasticity.

6. There is evidence, as presented above, that there are sufficient reasons to include pharmacotherapy in the treatment regime, or if it is suspected that the client's present prescription drugs may be causing unwanted side effects.

It is important to note that antidepressant medications can cause the activation of *latent psychosis*. This appears especially true of the tricyclic antidepressant medications, which may raise the level of catecholamines, including dopamine, which are excitatory neurotransmitters. It is well known that schizophrenia is exacerbated by rises in the levels of dopamine and norepinephrine, and this problem may extend to other forms of psychosis as well. This activation of latent psychosis is considered less likely for the nontricyclic antidepressant medications, particularly those that differentially raise serotonin levels (for example, sertraline [Zoloft] and fluoxetine [Prozac]).

COMPLIANCE.   Today, the number of depressed clients on antidepressant medications referred for psychothérapy is rising. Numerous reasons exist for this increase in antidepressant usage. Physicians who prescribe antidepressant medications are becoming better educated as to the drug-compliance and long-term recovery benefits to their patients of combining antidepressant medications and psychotherapy and therefore refer clients for counseling more readily. Given the reduced side effects (and lowered suicide risk) of the newer antidepressant medications (Prozac, Paxil, or Zoloft, for example), antidepressant medications are more likely to be prescribed for reactive depressive episodes. And physicians have a wider range of antidepressant medications to choose from when prescribing.

Counselors and other mental health workers need to be aware of clients' thinking processes that may affect their drug compliance. For example, clients often misattribute symptoms of their depressive illness to side effects of their antidepressant medication. This misattribution can lead to noncompliance and premature discontinuation of their medication. Rollman et al. (1996) suggest keeping very close check with clients about the entire range of their symptomatology prior to beginning and during application of the medication regime. Establishing a pretreatment baseline of symptoms will increase awareness of differences between depressive symptoms and drug side effects. This understanding may lead to better management of the treatment process.

Clients not thoroughly educated on the issues of medication therapy may believe that because they are in psychotherapy they are no longer expected to continue their antidepressant. Further, depressed clients' thinking and listening processes concerning their medications may be distorted by their depression; thus, clients may not process clearly what is said to them. Finally, clients may be entering psychotherapy as an alternative to drug therapy without having discussed discontinuing their medications with their prescribing physician. Let us look at the following case.

CASE HISTORY

Jan, a 25-year-old medical records coordinator for a local hospital, came to individual therapy on referral from her relationship-group facilitator. With signed consent, a review of Jan's progress notes from her group by a therapist under my supervision indicated a variety of relationship difficulties, somatic complaints, eating disorder, and a tentative (Rule Out: RO) diagnosis by her group leader of passive-aggressive personality disorder. A close reading of notes describing Jan's group behavior during the first five weeks of a 15-week group indicated an excessive concern with self-control and image management, determination to be thought well of by the group with intense aggressive displays when confronted by group members, and, finally, withdrawal from interaction. Rather than strengthening her social adaptation, Jan appeared to her group leader to be losing ground by coming to see herself in a more negative light. She also related to other group members in a more passive and self-deprecating manner. Although her Beck Depression Inventory (BDI) score continued to indicate mild depression, Jan began to express growing hopelessness and helplessness.

Individual therapy was recommended as a compliment to group, rather than a replacement. Jan presented to individual assessment as a very overweight young woman who, with an undergraduate degree in chemistry, was not working to her professional potential. Even though she had excellent grades, MEDCAT scores, and a father in the medical field, Jan had not been selected to attend medical school several years earlier. She spent her first session in therapy recounting her many interpersonal problems, family wrangling, career failures, and physical symptoms centered around PMS. During the first several supervision sessions, Jan was described by her therapist-in-training as whiny, irritating, a yes-but, and obsessed with control. Jan either told long-winded stories or sat silently. When confronted with feedback about her interpersonal style, Jan alternately cried and self-deprecated or criticized her therapist for being like those in her group who did not understand her. A bright young woman, however, Jan made some progress in understanding how her perfectionistic expectations were contributing to her problems. Not only could *she* not meet her expectations, she had applied them to others, who also failed to meet them and, thus, failed her as well. Jan continued to work on a variety of inter- and intrapersonal problems with growing insight into the nature of her difficulties.

Interestingly, however, even though her insight improved, Jan did not seem to improve in the group sessions (members felt she was passively sandbagging them and judging them), and, over time, she became less expressive during individual therapy, more dependent on the therapist, and more socially isolated in her new apartment away from her family.

Jan's therapist attributed her lack of progress to a variety of factors, including personality disorder (even though no etiological substructure for such a DSM Axis II diagnosis had been reasonably laid), lack of identity development (even though Jan's attachment background appeared adequate into young adulthood—her parents were busy and a bit intrusive but not overly controlling or abusive), and even malingering (even though little case had been made for secondary gain).

When asked how she felt when dealing with Jan, her therapist indicated that she felt depressed. "Exactly," I said, "That appears to me on videotape how your client feels! Even though her Beck Depression Inventory does not indicate severe depression, your client appears *very* depressed. She may be indicating it to you through parallel process (evoking her symptoms in her therapist and group) rather than through words." I advised my counselor-in-training that if her client continued with little improvement after a reassessment of the problem and an active approach to depression management, she should consider a referral for physical/psychiatric evaluation with a psychiatrist.

This advice was upsetting for the counselor for several reasons. First, she felt that it was indicative of a failure on her part to provide adequate therapy. Second, she had strong opinions about psychiatric medications for emotional problems (including depression), explaining that she believed they act as restraints (emotional brakes) on the one hand (a view that developed while working with chronically mentally ill patients during her externship at an inpatient psychiatric hospital) and are a "cheap fix" for a deeper problem on the other. I encouraged the counselor to more deeply explore the client's depressive symptomatology, to develop a more active depression-management plan, and to read more exhaustively in the area of medication management for depression.

As she followed these suggestions over several weeks, it became clearer to both client and counselor how her depression was interfering with her life. The client admitted being less than truthful about her depressive symptoms on the BDI for several reasons. First, several members of her family who struggled with depression (one with bipolar disorder) and alcoholism were avoided by her immediate family. These family members were considered the sick group from the client's perspective, and she did not want to be identified with them. One of Jan's uncles was bipolar and took lithium, and one suffered from alcoholism and depression and took antidepressants. Neither appeared, however, to be complying with their medication regime, and both had many hospitalizations. Second, her father, a physician, held strong negative opinions about psychiatric problems in general and psychiatric medications specifically, even though he had little formal training in this rapidly growing and complex area. The client stated that she had long been afraid that she would be prescribed medication for her problem (which she traced far back into adolescence with the help of her counselor), that her family, who were helping her with her bills, would find out, and that she would never be allowed to attend medical school in the future if it was discovered that she had taken psychiatric medications.

Even though Jan worked seriously on her depressive symptoms, she continued to be excessively irritable, self-focused and hopeless, unable to maintain a constant weight, or get restorative sleep. She found it more and more difficult to get up in the morning. She sometimes found herself sleeping on the job and feeling numb and dumb. Her interaction with friends became more constricted, and she talked about dropping out of her relationship group.

Importantly, and over a relatively short span of counseling (four sessions), Jan's counselor expressed higher and higher levels of irritation and a deepening sense of failure. During the fifth session, Jan told her surprised counselor that a friend had accompanied her to the hospital over the weekend due to some suicidal ideation that frightened Jan and her friend and that she had seen a psychiatrist who, after a thorough assessment, had prescribed an antidepressant medication (Zoloft) and encouraged Jan to continue with psychotherapy. Jan spent most of the next two sessions working on issues around telling her parents about her condition. She said that she did not expect the medication to help but thought, as a last resort, she would give it a try to help mediate her hopelessness. After about two weeks and, again, much to the surprise of her counselor, Jan began to work harder in therapy, making the most progress in her understanding of how she was exacerbating her interpersonal difficulties with her family and her group. She also reported having more energy, better sleep, less fatigue, and fewer angry withdrawal episodes in group. Over successive weeks, Jan reported that her weight was more stable, she had no further suicidal ideation, and she had decided to reapply to medical school in the spring.

Therapy with Jan took on a different tenor for the therapist, who became less self-blaming about her difficulties with Jan. Supervision indicated that her counselor was working more effectively with Jan on developing cognitive behavioral interventions for her interpersonal reticence and learned helplessness. The therapist was also able to confront Jan more directly about her many irrational and self-defeating beliefs. She helped Jan develop more creative solutions to a number of family and occupational problems and began, herself, to use a more interpersonal style of intervention with Jan as their relationship deepened. Interestingly, the therapist had to be reminded to check with Jan about her compliance with her medication regimen because, once therapy began to take a more positive shape, both the client and the therapist quickly began to attribute the therapist's success with her client to their interpersonal work together. Therapists, quite naturally I believe, make many false or "loaded" attributions: First, they believe that too much of the positive or negative variance in the client's condition is attributable to their interpersonal influence; second, and granted that client's must learn how to take responsibility for themselves, they attribute too much of the variance around the client's depression to the client's thinking processes and environmental factors. In many cases, endogenous or biological factors (hormonal changes, hypothyroidism coupled with dysthymia in Jan's case, for example) initiate cognitive and emotional distortion and lead to interpersonal and occupational problems. These social difficulties further exacerbate a physical deconditioning of the body, making it more vulnerable to somatic complaints. Social isolation further complicates the depressive cycle. It is often difficult to know what initiated the depressive cycle. The primary tip-off, about which counselors and supervisors must stay aware, is: when therapy languishes, the system must be entered through new means, including referral for psychiatric evaluation if clients become more hopeless after a reasonable application of therapy interventions and/or develop suicidal ideation or gestures. Referral for psychiatric evaluation is not a failure of therapy or therapist or client. It should be, rather, a proactive decision made by client and therapist together to further evaluate the etiological and consequential basis of the problem(s). Depression is often a cyclical biological-thinking-feeling-social/environmental system, which can be attacked from a variety of directions. The cycle can be broken over the long run, however, through concerted pressure at each point in the system. Clients must learn to address the cognitive, emotive, and behavioral facets of the problem as they arise, acknowledging that each facet may reemerge as different stresses develop.

Several important issues distinguish Jan's case: First, clients will often minimize their depressive symptoms in order to protect their families from embarrassment or financial costs and to please their therapists, who want to believe that their therapy is the answer to their clients' problems. Second, counselors tend to believe that therapy alone *should* be sufficient for their clients unless they are personality disordered or malingering. Third, counselors and clients are often untrained in understanding how psychiatric medications act as an adjunct to therapy by helping the client gain a foothold in therapy and speeding up the therapeutic process. Fourth, *supervisors* often misattribute clients' failure to stabilize in therapy to difficulties with their supervisees rather than encourage reassessment and possible referral; that is, supervisors may take too much responsibility for their counselors' progress rather than encourage a reevaluation of the client.

Box 2-3 provides a list of situations that may provide the base for a decision to reevaluate and refer. In the preceding case, the following red-flag conditions were emphasized: memory impairment, history of family member who has responded to antidepressant medication (uncle), history of family member with bipolar illness (uncle), presence of severe somatic complaints (PMS and other hormonal irregularities), partial (or poor) response to trial of cognitive therapy alone, historical evidence of chronic maladaptive functioning with depressive syndrome on an intermittent basis (R/O dysthymia in Jan's case), hopelessness, impaired concentration, severe depression with suicidal danger, and history of mania in a close relative.

CLASSES OF ANTIDEPRESSANTS

TRICYCLIC ANTIDEPRESSANTS

All **tricyclic antidepressants (TCAs)** have the same basic three-ring chemical structure and are related to the phenothiazine class of antipsychotics (Olin et al., 1998). TCAs are 65–75% effective in relieving the somatic features associated with depression, and TCAs have been shown to be effective in treating both exogenous and endogenous depression (Joyce & Paykel, 1989). TCAs are often prescribed for patients with decreased appetite, weight loss, early morning awakening, lack of interest in the people and objects in their environment, and a family history of depression combined with a history of responsiveness to medication. Conversely, highly anxious, fearful, or phobic patients who have many physical complaints and who have not improved with an adequate trial of TCAs may respond to monoamine oxidase inhibitors or second-generation antidepressant medications. It should be remembered that response to TCAs may differ by gender, although data on gender differences in response to TCAs is conflicting. Even though a majority of TCAs are taken by women, most clinical trials have utilized male subjects (Dawkins & Potter, 1991).

MECHANISMS AND ACTIONS.   TCA drugs exert their effects by blocking the reuptake of the excitatory neurotransmitters norepinephrine, dopamine, and 5-HT to the presynaptic membrane. Blocking the reuptake of these neurotransmitters causes an increase in the synaptic cleft. This blockade takes place through the medium of down-regulating receptors on the presynaptic membrane that provide information about decreasing transmitter release and/or rising reuptake levels. Secondarily, the TCAs also block postsynaptic receptors for acetylcholine and histamine, which accounts for their anticholinergic effects, including dryed mucus membranes and drowsiness (Julien, 1998). One TCA, clomipramine (Anafranil) specifically prevents the reuptake of 5-HT but not NE (Trimble, 1990), which accounts for its being the only TCA typically used for obsessive-compulsive disorder (OCD; Olin et al., 1998). Specific effects of TCAs include:

- mood elevation
- increase in physical activity and mental alertness
- improvement in sleep and appetite and
- nonelevation of mood in nondepressed subjects (American Medical Association, 1983)

PHARMACOKINETICS.   TCAs are easily absorbed and are not affected by the intake of food. Because most TCAs have long elimination half-lives (the time it takes the body to excrete one-half of the drug), they can be administered once a day, usually at bedtime. Metabolism occurs in the liver, and TCAs are excreted in the feces and urine. TCAs are highly protein-bound and, being very lipid (fat) soluble, are easily distributed throughout the brain (Olin et al., 1998).

DRUG INTERACTIONS.   Because they bind to plasma proteins in the bloodstream, TCAs increase the risk of interactions with other drugs. These interactions can be severe, especially in the geriatric population, who often take a wide range of medications, including OTCs. Drug interactions occur most frequently with drugs having sedative (benzodiazepine), anticholinergic (antihistamine), or hypotensive (blood pressure lowering) properties (Baldessarini, 1993).

SIDE EFFECTS.   Side effects are common with TCA therapy. However, a tolerance for anticholinergic medications usually develops over time. The most common side effects are the following:

- anticholinergic effects (especially common for people taking amitriptyline (Elavil) or imipramine (Tofranil) include dry mouth (50–74%), blurred vision (6–20%), urinary retention, and constipation
- cardiac arrhythmias
- hypertension—especially common among those taking Elavil or Tofranil sedation
- hypotension or dizziness (18–52%)
- other reversible side effects, such as seizures, insomnia, headache, tachycardia, tremor, and fatigue [Fuller & Underwood, 1989]

INTERACTIONS AND TOXICITY.   Because TCAs have a narrow therapeutic window, an acute overdose with TCAs can be fatal. With high doses, TCAs can produce serious hypotension (drop in blood pressure) that can lead to cardiac arrhythmia and death. Because these arrhythmias are very difficult to treat and because of the risk of TCA use in suicide, it is recommended that an acutely depressed or high-risk patient receive no more than a one-week supply of TCAs (Baldessarini, 1993).

DRUG SELECTION AND DOSING.   The selection of a specific TCA is based upon a patient's drug response history, target symptoms, and the TCA's side effects. Table 2-1 outlines the common uses of various TCAs. Dosages of TCAs are individualized. The initial dosage for a TCA is usually one-third to one-half of the therapeutic dose. If the desired response is not obtained, the dose is increased gradually. Gradual dose increases help minimize adverse effects (Swonger & Matejski, 1991). Response to the drug occurs within 14 to 21 days, with the maximum effect appearing in four to six weeks. TCA therapy is not considered ineffective until a four-week trial is completed with no measurable effects (Olin et al., 1998).

TCAs are not reinforcing drugs; they do not produce euphoria or stimulate the brain's pleasure centers. Because of the delay in the desired effects and the immediate appearance of side effects with TCAs, patients may become discouraged and discontinue treatment. It is imperative (a) that patients be encouraged to continue treatment until the medication has had a chance to work and (b) that patients be reassured that the usually bothersome anticholinergic side effects of TCAs do not usually impose serious problems and often abate within several weeks. Many anticholinergic side effects can also be controlled with Urecholine (bethanechol).

DISCONTINUATION.   Although TCAs are not addictive, abrupt discontinuation following a prolonged period of treatment can produce unwanted symptoms, including nausea, headache, vertigo, nightmares, and malaise. A gradual

Table 2-1   Tricyclic Antidepressants and Their Uses

Trade Name	Generic Name	Other Uses
Adapin	doxepin	Anxiety
		Chronic pain*
Anafranil	clomipramine	Only obsessive-compulsive disorders (OCD)
		Chronic pain*
		Panic disorder*
Asendin	amoxapine	
Aventyl	nortriptyline	Panic disorder*
Elavil	amitriptyline	Eating disorder*
		Chronic pain*
Endep	amitriptyline	Eating disorder*
		Chronic pain*
Norpramin	desipramine	Eating disorder* (bulimia)
		Facilitation of cocaine withdrawal*
Pamelor	nortriptyline	Panic disorder*
Pertofrane	desipramine	Eating disorder* (bulimia)
Sinequan	doxepin	Anxiety
		Chronic pain*
Surmontil	trimipramine	
Tofranil	imipramine	Child enuresis
		Panic disorder*
		Eating disorder* (bulimia)
Vivactil	protriptyline	

*Unlabeled use

Source: Olin et al., 1998.

withdrawal from the medication over two weeks will lessen these symptoms (Olin et al., 1998).

MONAMINE OXIDASE INHIBITOR ANTIDEPRESSANTS

Monoamine oxidase inhibitor antidepressants (MAOIs) are those that inhibit the actions of MAO, an enzyme that helps break down norepinephrine and serotonin and, therefore, increases NE and 5-HT in the synapse. MAOIs are indicated as treatment for depression in some patients who are unresponsive to other antidepressants. Due to their side-effects profile and the potential for serious interaction with other drugs and foods, irreversible MAOIs (those that bind irreversibly with MAO-A and MAO-B in tight chemical bonds) are rarely used first as the drug of choice when treating depression. Fortunately,

Table 2-2   MAOI Antidepressants and Their Uses

Trade Name	Generic Name	Other Uses
Marplan	isocarboxazid	
Nardil	phenelzine	Treatment-resistant
Parnate	tranylcypromine	Reactive depression

Source: Olin et al., 1998.

reversible MAOIs have recently been developed (brofaromine, pirlindole, toloxatone, and moclobimide) and because clinical trials are under way, should soon come into the marketplace.

The relationship between MAOIs and food intake stems from the regulation of tyramine metabolism by MAO. When MAO is inhibited, the presence of tyramine in the system can precipitate a hypertensive crisis (Julien, 1998). As we have said, MAOIs exert their effect by inhibiting the enzyme monoamine oxidase, which is responsible for the breakdown of the neurotransmitters norepinephrine (NE), serotonin (5-HT), and epinephrine, thereby increasing the levels of these neurotransmitters. The most common MAOIs are listed in Table 2-2. As with TCAs, there is usually a delay of several weeks in therapeutic action (Maxmen, 1991).

SIDE EFFECTS.   Common side effects of nonreversible MAOIs are postural hypotension (fall in blood pressure on standing), dizziness, headache, insomnia, fatigue, and tremors. Serious effects of MAOIs include liver damage and hypertensive crisis resulting from synergy with certain drugs and foods (Olin et al., 1998). This hypertension can be fatal, causing hemorrhaging in the brain. Reversible MAOIs have a much less difficult side-effect profile (little anticholinergic action) and interact very little with tyramine in food. They also appear to improve attention and memory somewhat among depressed clients (Julien, 1998).

DRUG INTERACTIONS AND TOXICITY.   Many over-the-counter (OTC) products, such as cold and sinus medicines, including those with dextromethorphan, present a serious hazard to patients taking irreversible MAOIs. The following are other drugs and foods that pose a serious threat if administered with or within two weeks of MAOI therapy.

Drugs to Avoid When Taking MAOIs—Foods to Avoid When Taking MAOIs

TCAs and other AMs	cheese	wine
Demerol (meperidine)	yogurt	beer
amphetamine stimulants	chocolate	cream
sympathomimetics	caffeine	pickled herring
tryptophan	fava beans	chicken liver

Table 2-3   Tetracyclic Antidepressants and Their Uses

Trade Name	Generic Name	Other Uses
Desyrel	trazadone	Cocaine withdrawal*
Ludiomil	maprotiline	Anxiety associated with depression
Remeron	mirtazapine	
*Unlabeled use		

Source: Olin et al., 1998.

Because of possible toxic and synergistic interactions with other antidepressants, MAOIs should be allowed sufficient time to clear the system before other antidepressant medications are begun. In some cases, this clearing period lasts four weeks in both directions—that is, MAOI cleared for non-MAOI, and non-MAOI cleared for use of MAOI.

TETRACYCLIC, SEROTONIN-SPECIFIC REUPTAKE INHIBITORS (SSRIS), AND MISCELLANEOUS ANTIDEPRESSANTS

The groups of newer antidepressants, sometimes referred to as **second generation**, and including tetracyclic, serotonin-specific (or selective serotonin) reuptake inhibitors and unrelated (or atypical) antidepressants, are usually contrasted with the tricyclics or first generation antidepressant medications. Tables 2-3, 2-4, and 2-5 list these antidepressants and their uses.

SSRIs and other second-generation antidepressants are somewhat less toxic and have a more rapid onset than tricyclics. They also produce fewer side effects, especially anticholinergic effects. As a general rule, the newer antidepressants produce less weight gain and less sedation and hypotension and

Table 2-4   Selective Serotonin Reuptake Inhibitor Antidepressants

Trade Name	Generic Name	Other Uses
Luvox	fluvoxamine	OCD
		Depression*
		PTSD
		Panic disorder
Paxil	paroxetine	OCD
		Panic disorder
		Headache*
Prozac	fluoxetine	Bulimia
		OCD
Zoloft	sertraline	OCD
*Unlabeled use		

Source: Olin et al., 1998.

Table 2-5   Atypical or Unrelated Antidepressants

Trade Name	Generic Name	Other Uses
Buspar	buspirone	Anxiety
Effexor	venlaxafine	
Meridia*	sibutramine	Obesity
Serzone	nefazadone	
Wellbutrin	bupropion	
Zyban	bupropion	Smoking cessation

*Not yet released

Source: Olin et al., 1998.

are potentially useful in treating obsessive-compulsive (repetitive or stereo-type) symptoms and eating disorders (McBride et al., 1991).

The second-generation antidepressant medications also produce their effects by raising levels of serotonin or up-regulating serotonin-2 receptors (5-HT2). Raising levels of 5-HT lowers depression in several important ways, including:

- inhibiting stimulation of areas in the limbic system that produce emotional pain reactions
- helping control obsessive rumination
- aiding in establishing proper sleep/awake cycles
- suppressing long-term, low-level pain transmission
- having important antianxiety effects
- acting to regulate or modulate other neurotransmitters responsible for alertness (NE, for example; Beasley, Masica, & Potvin, 1992; Delgado et al., 1991; Jonas & Schaumburg, 1991; Stahl, 1992).

CHARACTERISTICS OF SEROTONIN-SPECIFIC OR SELECTIVE REUPTAKE INHIBITORS (SSRIs)

The introduction of SSRIs, which are safer and have fewer side effects than, for example, TCAs and MAOIs, resulted in more frequent treatment of depression with medication. Table 2-4 lists the SSRIs and their uses. Because SSRIs are less lethal when taken in an overdose and because cardiac and anticholinergic side effects associated with tricyclic antidepressants are less dramatic, the SSRIs are considered safer for medically ill patients (Stoudemire, 1995). All SSRIs can produce dizziness or drowsiness, however, and caution is recommended when driving or performing tasks requiring alertness. Because of its sedative and synergistic effects, alcohol consumption (and any nonprescribed depressant medication) should be avoided. Another warning associated with SSRIs relates to their tendency to cause photosensitivity when exposed to the sun, and sunscreens are advised when taking an SSRI. Also, while advantageous to some,

SSRIs' effect of appetite suppression may be detrimental to others, especially for underweight clients (Olin et al., 1998).

SSRIs exert their effects by inhibiting the reuptake of serotonin in the neuron, which increases serotonin's activity in the brain. Again, some affect up- and down-regulation of autoreceptors on the presynaptic membrane, while some have the postsynaptic membrane as their primary seat of activity. It is important, because of the multiple ways they affect transmission through the synapses, to realize that when SSRIs are taken with other drugs (see the following list) they also can directly or indirectly elevate serotonin and serious problems can result. "Serotonin syndrome," an unwanted phenomenon represented by problems in cognition and in the autonomic and neuromuscular nervous systems, is a potentially life-threatening condition. There is no definitive test for serotonin syndrome, which may be caused by an up-regulation of the 5-HT receptors, and diagnosis is based on strong clinical suspicion. It is common for the earliest symptoms to be mistaken as a worsening of the patient's psychiatric condition (Tornatore, 1996). Clients and patients whose condition worsens appreciably after prescription of antidepressants should be encouraged to contact their physician. Keeping close track of the client's complete medication regimen, especially focusing on the addition or subtraction of drugs, whether or not they are OTC, is imperative in working with clients on psychiatric medications.

Drug Combinations Associated with Serotonergic Syndrome
- MAOIs with SSRIs, meperidine (Demerol), or dextromethorphan
- Fenfluramine component in Fen/Phen and dexfenfluramine (Redux) with SSRIs or MOAIs
- Lithium combined with other serotonergic agents (Tornatore, 1996)

A CLOSER LOOK AT SELECTED SSRIs

CELEXA (CITALOPRAM).   Celexa is a selective serotonin reuptake inhibitor (SSRI) that is not closely related to other SSRIs or the TCAs. It is reported to have minimal effects on norepinephrine and dopamine uptake. So far around 8 million patients around the world have received citalopram, which was marketed first in Denmark in 1989. Celexa is reported to have a favorable side-effect profile, with mild anticholinergic effects. As with most therapeutic drugs, alcohol and other drugs that affect the central nervous system, including other antidepressants (especially MAOIs), should be discontinued while Celexa is being taken.

LUVOX (FLUVOXAMINE).   Fluvoxamine appears to be as effective in treating depression as the TCAs. Its mode of action is the reduction of serotonin turnover. It appears to positively affect obsessive-compulsive syndromes, possibly through autoreceptor desensitization. Like other antidepressant medications, fluvoxamine may provoke mania in some bipolar clients. Common side effects include headache, nausea, vomiting, diarrhea, insomnia, excessive sleepiness, dizziness, and agitation (Olin et al., 1998; Guthrie et al., 1996). These side effects usually remit within several weeks.

PAXIL (PAROXETINE). Paroxetine was introduced in early 1993 and has become a first-line medication. Other uses now include OCD and panic disorder. Like sertraline and fluoxetine, it exerts its action by inhibiting serotonin reuptake, thereby increasing the amount of serotonin in the synapse. Paroxetine can be given once daily, usually in the morning. The initial dose is 20 mg per day and can be increased to 50 mg daily. Similar to all antidepressants, the full therapeutic effect may be delayed. Side effects are relatively mild and are dose related. Patients usually develop tolerance to its adverse effects (Olin et al., 1998).

PROZAC (FLUOXETINE). Fluoxetine is now the most frequently prescribed antidepressant, with more than 800,000 prescriptions written each month during the early 1990s (Jonas & Schaumburg, 1991). Many more prescriptions are currently written, and it is a first-line antidepressant. In addition to major depression, other FDA-approved uses for Prozac include bulimia nervosa and OCD. Research shows that for most people fluoxetine has fewer side effects than TCAs, producing a less "drugged" feeling. Fluoxetine accomplishes its antidepressant effect by raising levels of the neurotransmitter serotonin (5-HT) by decreasing its reuptake by the presynaptic membrane of the neuron; slowed reuptake is thought to be primarily accomplished by down-regulation of presynaptic inhibitory autoreceptors (Beasley et al., 1992). It also appears to differentially affect 5-HT2 receptors believed to be particularly important in the regulation of mood.

Side effects and drug interactions. Fluoxetine has endured great controversy. Claims against fluoxetine, which are based on anecdotal evidence, have associated its use with acts of violence and suicide (Beasley et al., 1991). However, the FDA has ruled that fluoxetine should be kept on the market because its low risk of associated paradoxical effects appears no greater than risks associated with other antidepressant medications. The National Mental Health Association and a variety of others have maintained that fluoxetine is extremely useful in treating depression.

Recommendations are to begin with a dose of 20 mg in the morning. If no improvement is noticed within several weeks, the dose is increased. Full antidepressant effects may be delayed until four weeks. Finally, although drinking alcohol should be firmly discouraged because it is often addictive and certainly exacerbates depression, fluoxetine has very low levels of interaction with alcohol (Jonas & Schaumburg, 1991). At the time of this writing, only two deaths from an overdose of fluoxetine have been reported; autopsies on both cases indicated that other drugs were involved. Common side effects include decrease in appetite, shakiness, dizziness, nervousness, insomnia, and decrease in libido. Clients should not suddenly discontinue Prozac without their physicians' guidance (Olin et al., 1998).

ZOLOFT (SERTRALINE).   Sertraline is structurally quite similar to fluoxetine and its antidepressant actions are also due to the inhibition of 5-HT reuptake. Zoloft, approved for marketing in December 1991, is also used for treatment of OCD, and its effects may be delayed by several weeks. Side effects noted with Zoloft include headaches, dizziness, nausea, restlessness, sleeplessness, dry mouth, and increased sweating (Olin et al., 1998).

MISCELLANEOUS AND SPECIAL USE ANTIDEPRESSANTS

ANAFRANIL (CLOMIPRAMINE).   Clomipramine (see Table 2-1) is a TCA that restricts serotonin reuptake and, probably due to that quality, has been used specifically for the treatment of OCD. About 50% of patients with OCD respond favorably, particularly when Anafranil is used in conjunction with behavior therapy; Anafranil has been used in the United States since 1990 but has been used in Canada and Europe for many years. It has also been used successfully in the treatment of panic and phobic disorders, as well as depression (Julien, 1998).

BUSPAR (BUSPIRONE).   Buspirone (see Table 2-5) is a selective serotonin (5-HT sub-1A) receptor agonist or enhancer. It is used primarily in the treatment of anxiety; however, research has also found that Buspar, like other 5-HT partial agonist drugs, does have some antidepressant effects. These antianxiety and antidepressant properties are contradictory and are usually explained in the following way. As a partial agonist, buspirone or gepirone would compete with an oversupply of 5-HT, thus reducing its effects and acting as a functional antagonist. However, in depression (a deficiency of 5-HT) the drug's agonist properties would, first, allow the presynaptic membrane to replenish serotonin stores and, second, act as an agonist at the postsynaptic receptor in the condition of deficit 5-HT, which would cause a rise in activity and, thus, raise depression. Adjunctive use with other antidepressants is not fully researched (Napoliello & Domantay, 1991; Olin et al., 1998).

DESYREL (TRAZODON).   Trazodon (see Table 2-3) is a tetracyclic AM that is structurally unique. Its mode of action, which is not fully understood, appears to be the blockade or down-regulation of 5-HT2 and NE receptors. Its use in males is somewhat limited due to the risk of priapism, sustained and painful erection, which may be due to its down-regulation of NE. It is sometimes prescribed to persons withdrawing from cocaine (Olin et al., 1998) and produces moderate sedation.

EFFEXOR (VENLAFAXINE).   Venlafaxine was approved for treatment of depression in late 1993. It is structurally unique and blocks the reuptake of norepinephrine as well as serotonin, and it resembles fluoxetine in character. Because of it's short half-life, Effexor requires multiple daily dosing, but its primary metabolite is active for over 10 hours. Side effects include nervousness, sweating, and decrease in appetite (which appear related to its blockade of NE), dizziness, and minimal dry mouth (Stoudemire, 1995).

LUVOX (FLUVOXAMINE).   Fluvoxamine (see Table 2-4) is an SSRI with few TCA side effects, particularly cardiac, and is comparable in effect with imipramine. Compared with other SSRIs, Luvox appears to be more useful in the treatment of PTSD, dysphoria, and panic disorder (Julien, 1998). However, direct comparisons with many other SSRIs have not been conducted and caution is warranted in comparing the efficacy of SSRIs in a variety of treatment domains.

MERIDIA (SIBUTRAMINE).   Sibutramine (see Table 2-5) inhibits the reuptake of serotonin, norepinephrine, and possibly dopamine (Olin et al., 1998). This medication is currently undergoing trials for the treatment of depression and obesity. Side effects include increases in blood pressure that may reflect its blockade of reuptake of NE and DA and increase risk of cardiac toxicity.

SERZONE (NEFAZODONE).   In 1994, Serzone (see Table 2-5) was approved for use in depressive illnesses. It has dual 5-HT actions, including blockade of 5-HT2A receptors (which helps explain its positive effects on sleep and anxiety and the lack of increased sexual dysfunction), and inhibits serotonin reuptake (which explains its antidepressant action; Guthrie et al., 1996).

WELLBUTRIN (BUPROPION).   Because of the possibility of seizures, alcohol consumption is ill advised when taking bupropion (see Table 2-5). Levodopa and MAOIs should also be avoided. Motor coordination may be impaired with its use. Common adverse effects include headache, dry mouth, constipation, sweating, dizziness, tremors, and insomnia (Olin et al., 1998). An advantage is that Wellbutrin causes little or no sexual dysfunction (Saklad, 1997). Wellbutrin exerts its effects by inhibiting dopamine reuptake (Ferris, Cooper, & Maxwell, 1983), a mechanism similar to that of stimulant drugs (cocaine) and, secondarily, by inhibiting turnover (reuptake) of norepinephrine. Several of its metabolites also appear to have antidepressant properties (Goodnick, 1991). Bupropion's potential for abuse is unclear. It has been used in the treatment of cocaine abuse, Parkinson's disease, and chronic fatigue syndrome without significant adverse reactions (Goodnick, 1991). In 1997, Wellbutrin's manufacturer received approval for marketing bupropion under the name of Zyban, which has been proven effective in smoking cessation. Also, at that time, Wellbutrin SR, a sustained-release formulation, was introduced. Both Zyban and Wellbutrin SR have the advantages of less frequent dosing and, theoretically, a better side-effect profile (less gastrointestinal disturbance and less insomnia; Saklad, 1997).

CHARACTERISTICS OF TETRACYCLIC ANTIDEPRESSANTS

Table 2-3 lists the three common tetracyclic antidepressants (Desyrel, Ludiomil, and Remeron) and their uses. Although their exact mechanism of action is unknown, it is postulated that these drugs increase serotonergic and noradrenergic activity in the brain. Collectively, these drugs have a lower incidence of anticholinergic side effects. However, their central nervous system side effects—drowsiness, dizziness, and impairment of cognitive and motor skills—warrant caution. Due to its sedative effects, Deseryl (trazadone) is often prescribed in conjunction with other antidepressants as a sleep aide (see "Drug Combinations Used in Depression"), while Remeron may produce an increase or decrease in appetite (Olin et al., 1998).

DRUG COMBINATIONS USED IN DEPRESSION

Due to the numerous variables in clients' genetic makeup and lifestyle and the many variations of depressive illnesses, discovering the perfect antidepressant is a great challenge. Often, psychiatrists prescribe more than one antidepressant (at the same time) for a client. An example of this practice is L.G., a 42-year-old black female who had been depressed. Originally, she was given Zoloft (sertraline) and responded positively to treatment as evidenced by brighter mood and more hopeful outlook. However, she expressed concern to her doctor because it was becoming increasingly more difficult to fall asleep. Her sleep problems led to daytime drowsiness and an increase in anxiety relating to fears of relapse. L.G.'s doctor addressed this problem by augmenting her Zoloft with Deseryl (Trazadone). Within a week of the addition of Deseryl, L.G.'s sleep improved and anxiety remitted.

Another combination used in treatment of depression involves the use of an SSRI, such as Zoloft, with Neurontin (gabapentin). Similar to Deseryl, Neurontin helps induce restorative sleep. Psychiatrists have also met with some success in prescribing small doses of antipsychotics with antidepressants for depressed patients with borderline personality disorder. Consider the case of Rachel, a 27-year-old female. Rachel had a significant history of abuse and had been engaged in treatment for a few years. After numerous episodes of instability and subsequent hospitalizations, Rachel's psychiatrist prescribed a small dose of Stelazine (an antipsychotic) alongside Prozac (an antidepressant). Her doctor and her counselor noted improvements in her functioning as evidenced by fewer crises and a reduction in suicidal ideation. Psychiatrists have also noted positive results when prescribing small doses of Zyprexa (a new antipsychotic agent discussed briefly later) to augment the effects of antidepressants.

DUAL-ACTION ANTIDEPRESSANTS

All psychotropic medications affect multiple sites in the brain and a number of different receptors for various neurotransmitters. Most produce a variety of types of symptom relief. Serzone (nefazodone) and Remeron (miretazapine) have been called *dual-action antidepressants* because of the range of their therapeutic action. By 5-HT2A receptor blockade, Serzone is beneficial for sleep and anxiety without inducing sexual dysfunction. By its actions to block serotonin reuptake, it acts as an antidepressant. Thus, it appears to be as effective as other antidepressants and has fewer negative side effects than most antianxiety medications while acting as an **anxiolytic**.

Remeron also functions as an antidepressant, through enhancing NE and 5-HT activity, while at the same time preventing side effects common to SSRIs, including anxiety, insomnia, agitation, nausea, and sexual dysfunction (Julien, 1998). Other drugs that could be considered dual-action antidepressants include some of the drugs used in the treatment of psychosis, including risperidone (Risperdal), olanzapine (Zyprexa), and sertindole (Serlect), which appear to be effective in relieving not only many of the positive (psychotic features) but many negative (often depressive) symptoms of schizophrenia as well.

TREATMENT RESPONSE.   A poorer response to medication is predicted for individuals who have experienced an abrupt onset to depression and have a history of depressive episodes that are of long duration. Biological and situational depressions appear to respond similarly to medication, especially the vegetative, somatic symptoms. However, severe melancholic depressions do respond better to some antidepressive medications than others, particularly bupropion (Wellbutrin) and nortriptyline (Pamelor, a TCA, see Table 2-1) and electroconvulsive therapy (ECT) as opposed to serotonin-selective reuptake inhibitors (SSRIs; *Psychopharmcology Update*, July 1998; see Tables 2-4 and 2-5). Although psychotherapy is thought to affect most cognitive and emotional symptoms, the effects of antidepressant medications on mood and emotional symptoms should not be underestimated. Emotional pain is caused by changes in neurotransmission, particularly in the hypothalamus, not simply by painful thoughts.

Two of the most commonly prescribed antidepressant medications (tricyclics; see Table 2-1), amitriptyline (Elavil) and imipramine (Tofranil), are more likely to raise blood pressure. Thus, if clients have hypertension, either doxepin (Sinequan), a tricyclic antidepressant with low hypertensive qualities, or a second generation AM may be prescribed. Counselors should be reminded that idiosyncratic (out-of-the-ordinary), paradoxical (reversed), toxic, and allergic reactions can occur with all drugs. Ask the client to arrange to have a medication evaluation if acute physical or divergent psychiatric problems persist.

DEPRESSION IN THE ELDERLY

Age and depression are highly and positively correlated, and this is particularly true when social attachments deteriorate among the aging (Mullins &

Dugan, 1991; Plotkin, Gerson, & Jarvik, 1987). Age-related depressive effects include decreased metabolic activity, cerebral blood flow, oxygen metabolism, and neurotransmitter concentrations (Busse & Simpson, 1983; Yesavage, 1992). Five million of the 33 million older adults (65 years or older) suffer from serious and persistent symptoms of depression, while 1 million have major depression (Saklad, 1997). Although the elderly represent only 12% of the population, they account for 20% of suicides (6000) each year (Yesavage, 1992). From 1980 to 1992, the suicide rate among the elderly increased by 9%, and among adults 85 years or older, the suicide rate increased by 35% (Saklad, 1997). Considering suicide rates in the elderly, less severe episodes of depression should not be regarded as normal and acceptable characteristics of the aging process. Early and appropriate attention to depression can decrease symptoms, decrease risk of recurrence, increase quality of life, improve medical health, decrease cost of health care, and decrease mortality. Even though many health problems, such as stroke, dementia, and Parkinson's disease, are usually accompanied by depressive episodes, rather than waiting until the somatic disorder improves, treatment for depression should be introduced once the diagnosis is made (Stovell, 1996).

Depression among the aged is often masked by or mistaken for physiological or other psychological problems. Physiological masks include loss of memory and concentration, gastrointestinal problems, poor overall health, arthritic changes, and heart disease (Yesavage, 1992), other medications, and drug abuse (Crook et al., 1987). Psychological problems that have a masking effect include anxiety, grief, insomnia, confusion, impulsivity, unwarranted anger, and apathy (Fredrick & Fredrick, 1985; Yesavage, 1992). Yesavage (1992) indicates that, contrary to common opinion, depressed geriatric clients *usually do not* have a long history of memory loss, disorientation, incontinence, neurological signs such as muscle weakness or **ataxia** (loss of coordination), or aphasia (loss of speech production facility or loss of social appropriateness). Further, they are usually oriented, even though they may be too angry to answer questions, and their cognitive problems are erratic rather than continuous.

All elderly clients need thorough assessment because of their heightened sensitivity to drugs and to social effects. The most effective forms of psychotherapy with the elderly emphasize reengaging the client (and spouse or family) in activities that will increase cognitive, emotional, and social-behavioral awareness and that rely on social (or institutional) support to decrease negative rumination and isolation (Busse & Simpson, 1983; Mullins & Dugan, 1991; Mishara & Kastenbaum, 1980).

Yesavage (1992) points out that if clients do not respond to psychotherapy they should certainly be referred for evaluation for antidepressant therapy. He also notes that the best antidepressant would be one that has few side effects, a short half-life, and few active metabolites and would induce few interactions with other drugs. Fortunately, although the tricyclic antidepressants do not fit this profile very well, the tetracyclics and SSRI antidepressant medications do

(Branconnier et al., 1983). Sertraline (Zoloft), for example, a serotonin-reuptake inhibitor, has low anticholinergic effects, low lethality on overdose, low sedation, a moderately short half-life, does not potentiate alcohol, and produces few drug interactions (Olin et al., 1998). It should be remembered that sensitivity to antidepressant medications, especially amitriptyline (a TCA), rises with age and that, therefore, smaller doses are more likely to be adequate for older clients. Antidepressant medications are also more likely, even at low doses, to produce interactions with other medications older adults may be taking (Dawkins & Potter, 1991).

NEW DIRECTIONS IN ANTIDEPRESSANT THERAPY

Researchers are developing antidepressants that affect only some of many serotonin receptors, with the goals of increased efficacy and fewer side effects ("New Drugs", 1998). Further, a new class of antidepressants under development would block yet another type of receptor site, the NK-1, and more drugs are being developed that affect both serotonin and norepinephrine or combinations of other neurotransmitter systems. Researchers and practitioners are trying more combined drug regimes. All these experiments involve efforts to better treat depressive symptoms, decrease unpleasant side effects, or both. Conversely, medications are being tested for breadth of clinical utility. For example, a study by Zenardi et al. (1996) found that SSRIs alone were effective for some clients with psychotic features accompanying their depression. As new medications continue to be developed at a rapid rate, you will likely find clients reporting medications not listed in your references. Pharmacists provide an excellent resource for information on new, as well as existing, drugs.

BIPOLAR AFFECTIVE DISORDER

Bipolar affective disorder, or simply bipolar disorder, is commonly referred to as manic-depression. Criteria established by the DSM-IV (APA, 1994) state that an individual must have at least one episode of mania and one of depression to be diagnosed with bipolar disorder. An accurate diagnosis may be difficult because approximately 30% of all patients having a manic episode experience hallucinations or delusions, which makes it difficult to separate bipolar disorder from schizophrenia or other psychosis-inducing illness. Unfortunately, where symptoms of bipolar disorder are confused with features of schizophrenia, misdiagnosis can lead to administration of inappropriate drug therapy, often for long periods of time.

Between 0.4 and 1.2% of the general population is affected by bipolar affective disorder, with males and females being equally affected (Rosenbaum, 1988). For diagnostic purposes, bipolar disorders are divided by DSM-IV (APA, 1994) into four categories:

1. Mixed (currently alternating mania and depression)
2. Manic (not currently depressed)
3. Depressed (not currently manic)
4. Cyclothymic (presence for at least two years of numerous hypomanic episodes interspersed with episodes of depression that do not meet the criteria for major depressive episodes)

Approximately 10% of the patients with bipolar affective disorder experience rapid cycling, which is defined as at least four illness episodes (of either mania or depression) within one year (Ellenor & Dishman, 1996). Rapid cyclers can move from depression to mania and back over a period as short as 24 hours. Clients with mixed bipolar affective disorder comprise 40% of those so diagnosed, and the mania experienced with the mixed form is characterized as more dysphoric than euphoric (Ellenor & Dishman, 1996).

ETIOLOGY

Bipolar disorder results from a chemical imbalance in the brain, not from sociological or interpersonal factors as is still believed too often today. Positron emission tomography (PET) scans show remarkable differences in brain activity between the manic and depressive cycles. The manic, hyperexcited phase is apparently brought on by a lack of reuptake of excitatory neurotransmitter NE into the presynaptic membrane. The depressive phase is thought to be brought on by exhaustion of the production of excitatory neurotransmitters, by changes in responsiveness of the receptors for these neurotransmitters, or by hormonal (or other neuromodulator) changes that are triggered by hyperexcitability (Julien, 1998; Lickey & Gordon, 1995). Both abnormal neurotransmitter activity and receptor responsiveness are noted in patients with manic-depression.

The occurrence of bipolar disorder is greatly influenced by genetics and, like unipolar depression, 60–80% of individuals with first-degree relatives who experience bipolar disorder will also experience some form of depressive syndrome (Restak, 1988). It is important for counselors to remember that clients' concerns about inheriting the disorder, or passing the disorder to their children, can themselves engender fear, hopelessness, and, at times, learned helplessness. This overriding concern may occur even within high-risk offspring to whom the syndromes have apparently *not* been transferred.

TREATMENT

Lithium was first used for treatment of mania in the 1940s. Since that time, it has been established that manic-depression is effectively controlled by administration of lithium in approximately 80% of cases with classic symptoms of manic-depression and with an acceptable side effect profile (Baldessarini, 1993). Fortunately, many who do not do well on lithium alone or present with more complex features, can be treated successfully with newer first-line agents (the second generation drugs for bipolar disorder), carbamazepine, and dival-proex sodium (Depakote) or with a combination of lithium and carbamazepine (Tegretol; Shukla & Cook, 1989). DSM IV lists several bipolar spectrum disorders, including Bipolar I, which is characterized by more prominent mania, and Bipolar II, which is characterized by major depressive and hypomanic episodes, and cyclothymia (subclinical depression and hypomania). Neurontin (gabapentin), and Lamotrigine, antiseizure medications, are often used if the first-line drugs are not fully successful (see Figures 2-1 and 2-2). Both have mood stabilizing and antidepressant effects and, therefore, are used with treatment-resistant patients. Both drugs are under consideration for approval by the FDA for use in bipolar disorders.

Carbamazepine, often in combination with other psychotropics, has also been used with various levels of success for a variety of Axis 1 and Axis 2 disorders, including, for example, affective disorders, impulse control disorders, PTSD, and some schizophrenia spectrum disorders (Julien, 1998). The older mood stabilizers such as lithium and valproic acid (Depakote or Depakene) appear to be more suitable for the manic component of bipolar disorder rather than depressive symptoms. However, when an antidepressant is added, the risks of inducing mania or rapid cycling of moods are an important consideration.

Approximately 40% of bipolar clients remain well after three years of drug treatment. This figure reflects the difficulties that clients have with side effects from lithium treatment, the seductive nature of the manic highs to which clients often wish a return, and difficulties making progress in psychotherapy. No studies support the effectiveness of psychotherapy alone for the treatment of bipolar affective disorder, and lithium has not been found to be effective with other forms of depression (Lickey & Gordon, 1995). Depression is often the more difficult part of the disorder to treat effectively over the long run. This finding highlights the importance of integrating psychotherapy, especially depression and behavior management, with drug therapy. Fortunately, patients in psychotherapy are more accepting of their diagnosis, more compliant with their prescriptions, and show added improvements in social and occupational functioning (Ellenor & Dishman, 1996).

Therapists are of great benefit to clients and their families in helping them understand the importance of day-to-day routine and in helping clients develop habits that promote medication compliance. There appears to be a "kindling" effect whereby successive episodes of depression or mania cause the brain to become more easily disregulated. Without proper treatment or with poor compliance, patients are likely to face a deteriorating course of the disease; therefore, the better regulated patients become and the fewer the episodes of mania and depression, the better the course of the disease process is likely to be.

Psychotherapy can help clients address the problems of living that often arise from bipolar affective disorder, even when cyclic episodes are under relatively adequate control. Unfortunately, those who suffer from bipolar illness

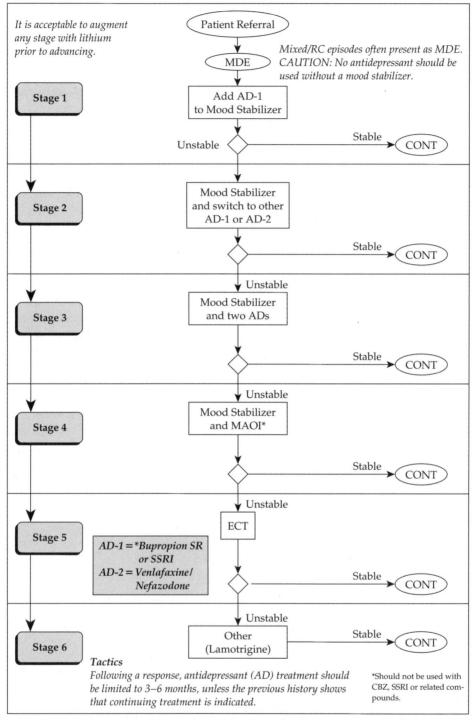

It is acceptable to augment any stage with lithium prior to advancing.

Patient Referral

MDE

Mixed/RC episodes often present as MDE. CAUTION: No antidepressant should be used without a mood stabilizer.

Stage 1

Add AD-1 to Mood Stabilizer

Unstable — Stable → CONT

Stage 2

Mood Stabilizer and switch to other AD-1 or AD-2

Stable → CONT

Unstable

Stage 3

Mood Stabilizer and two ADs

Stable → CONT

Unstable

Stage 4

Mood Stabilizer and MAOI*

Stable → CONT

Unstable

Stage 5

ECT

*AD-1 = *Bupropion SR or SSRI*
AD-2 = Venlafaxine/ Nefazodone

Stable → CONT

Unstable

Stage 6

Other (Lamotrigine)

Stable → CONT

Tactics
Following a response, antidepressant (AD) treatment should be limited to 3–6 months, unless the previous history shows that continuing treatment is indicated.

*Should not be used with CBZ, SSRI or related compounds.

Source: Bipolar Disorders Module: BPD Guideline Procedures Manual, Texas Medication Algorithm Project (TMAP), Texas Department of Mental Health and Mental Retardation, Austin, TX.

Figure 2-1 Strategies for the treatment of bipolar disorders: Major depressive episodes.

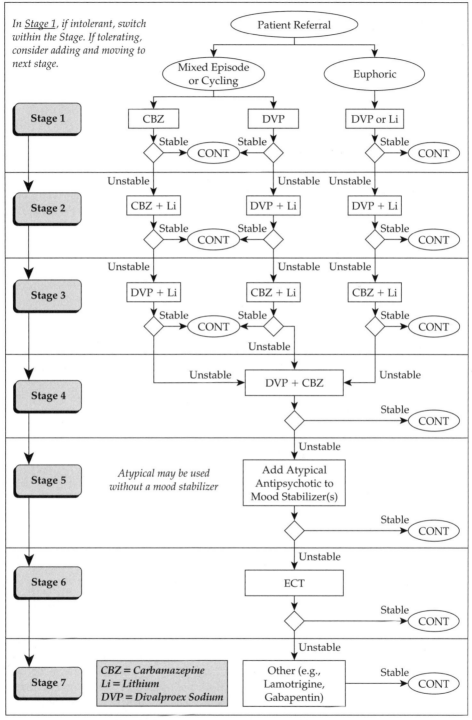

Source: Bipolar Disorders Module: BPD Guideline Procedures Manual, Texas Medication Algorithm Project (TMAP), Texas Department of Mental Health and Mental Retardation, Austin, TX.

Figure 2-2 Strategies for the treatment of bipolar disorders: Hypo-manic/manic episodes.

are poorly understood by the general public and, often, by their own families. Bipolar patients have long histories of rejection, relationship difficulties, and issues of self-esteem and self-efficacy.

Many who suffer from bipolar disorder, especially those who experience cycles of hypomania and then mild to moderate depression (cyclothymia), find it difficult to give up the highs, even though the lows are very painful. Cyclothymic individuals often discontinue their psychiatric medication(s) and sometimes medications for other medical conditions as well because they no longer experience their lives as creative, energetic, or fruitful or because they feel overwhelmed by the drug's early side effects. Fortunately, many clients with bipolar disorder find that their creativity and energy are not diminished over the long run, even though their disorganization and depression are controlled by the lithium medication. Men and women appear to react in much the same manner to lithium. Lithium treatment should be closely monitored or other drugs substituted if possible for pregnant women, however, because research reported by Dawkins and Potter (1991) indicates that malformations occurred in 11% of babies born to a sample of 225 women on lithium treatment.

During fully manic episodes, the client moves from feelings of extreme well-being, euphoria, control, and purpose to feelings of being inspired, all encompassing, all knowing, and omnipotent, while behaviorally growing more and more disorganized and impulsive. Particularly in the manic phase, but sometimes during depression, the patient may become psychotic, primarily delusional, even though hallucinations are not common.

CASE STUDY: BIPOLAR WITH PSYCHOTIC FEATURES

Margaret, a 22-year-old, single, British-American music student with a history of bipolar disorder arrived for outpatient family therapy. Margaret and her family related the following story:

FIRST MANIC EPISODE.   During spring semester, Margaret, then 19, stopped attending college for several weeks. She lay at home on the couch all day and responded irritably to family members. She denied using any drugs. Her parents attributed her behavior to adolescence and alternated between trying to talk with her and being highly critical. After a month, she began pacing for hours around the house and staying up all night watching movies. Margaret's mother took her to see their family physician when Margaret had been without sleep for about four days in a row. After ruling out a drug-induced mood disorder, the doctor diagnosed Margaret with having a bipolar disorder and prescribed lithium. Her parents did not believe that Margaret needed medication but reluctantly went along with the doctor's recommendation. Unfortunately, when Margaret soon ceased compliance with her drug regimen, they expressed their agreement with her decision. She returned to school in the fall and maintained average grades.

SECOND MANIC EPISODE.   About ten months after returning to school, Margaret disappeared for three days with the family car, and when she returned, she had driven over 2000 miles. She placed a sign in the yard that read "MARGARET MILLER HOME FROM GRAND TOUR." She had charged $1000 in food, gas, and motel fees on her trip. Initially, her father reacted angrily and made a list of strict rules for her to follow. Soon thereafter, Margaret took the car to the hardware store without permission and returned to find her father standing in the driveway yelling angrily at her. Margaret shouted back and began banging a shovel she had bought on the driveway cement. Neighbors called the police, who took Margaret into custody for a few hours and persuaded her parents to seek medical attention for their daughter.

Her parents took her back to their family physician, who restarted Margaret on lithium and referred Margaret to a psychiatrist. She did not see a psychiatrist and only took the lithium for a month. She stopped taking her lithium a second time because of her increasing weight (which is a side effect of lithium). Once again, her parents did not make efforts to help Margaret take her medication regularly or press her to keep an appointment for a psychiatric evaluation.

DEVELOPING BEHAVIOR PATTERNS.   Margaret then went through periods of functioning adequately and periods of irritability, poor sleep, and erratic behavior. Her mother admitted feeling nervous about her daughter's behavior at times but said she wrote it off to adolescence. Her father became very frustrated with her bouts of midnight pacing. He later said that she wore a rut around the outside of the house. He became angry with his wife and accused her of encouraging irresponsible behavior. He had high hopes for his daughter to be the first family member to graduate from college and believed her singing voice to be of professional quality. During her third manic episode, Margaret's mother observed that Margaret started eating only tuna fish and lettuce and declared all other foods poisonous. Margaret grew even more irritable and loud and spoke so rapidly everyone had trouble understanding her meaning. Her mother found a letter Margaret wrote to the police claiming her parents were trying to poison her. Margaret refused to go back to the doctor and refused to start taking the lithium again.

Margaret finally disappeared for 24 hours with the family car, and when she returned, her parents forced her to see a psychiatrist. During the psychiatric interview, Margaret conveyed no awareness that her behavior was anything out of the ordinary and explained matter-of-factly that her parents were making things up and they needed treatment, not her. The psychiatrist received her parents' permission to hospitalize Margaret in order to regulate her on medication.

In the hospital, Margaret received Depakote for her symptoms of mania and Risperdal for her distorted, paranoid thinking. She attended group, individual, and recreation therapy. As she became calmer, her speech assumed a normal rate and loudness. She spoke in a pleasant, matter-of-fact tone of voice. Staff did not encourage her in her efforts to talk about her delusions (e.g., that most food was poisonous). She ate a much wider variety of food than on admission, even though she still held irrational food beliefs. However, she continued to deny needing medication and did not develop insight into her illness.

Margaret experienced a brief setback when she secretly stopped taking her medication. Her hospital therapist found a letter written to an outside laboratory saying that the hospital staff was holding her prisoner and forced her to take poisons. Soon Margaret resumed the loud, demanding behavior and rapid speech she had exhibited on first hospitalization, and became less amenable to reason from hospital staff.

Her inpatient psychiatrist continued her on Risperdal and Depakote by mouth but with closer staff supervision. Soon Margaret regained therapeutic ground. Meanwhile, her parents began attending meetings of the local Alliance for the Mentally Ill, designed to help family members cope with the impact of mental illness on a loved one. They began reading about bipolar disorder and reading books by people living with the disease. On visits to the hospital, her father spoke less judgmentally about her past behavior. He began to understand it as part of a disease—something for Margaret to learn to manage, with the help of medication, psychotherapy, and family/social support, rather than warranting his punishment.

DISCHARGE PLANNING.   Just before discharge from the hospital during a family psycho-educational session, Margaret's parents talked about what they were learning and expressed a newfound belief that Margaret did indeed suffer from a mental illness and needed medication. Margaret had her own concerns. She asked that her parents be willing to attend outpatient family therapy with her, not to focus on her illness, but to work on family issues. She described her mother as very compliant and her father as very critical and as drinking beer daily to excess. Reflecting on a comment her father had made to her mother when he was drinking one night, Margaret asked rhetorically, "How can you stir soup wrong?" Margaret and her parents negotiated mutual commitments. Margaret agreed to let her parents watch her swallow her medication, which she still did not believe she needed. Her parents agreed to attend family therapy with her to work on family issues.

BEGINNING FAMILY THERAPY.   This request by Margaret highlights the importance of focusing on assessment, treatment, and education of the client's family. Family therapy requires special attention to establishing a safe environment and clear ground rules for communication. Structured formats for expressing strong emotions are necessary, along with a general de-emphasis on catharsis. Therapy should include teaching the family group problem solving, negotiating control contracts about commitments, and renegotiating commitments. Boszormenyi-Nagy and Krasner's (1986) discussion of family loyalties and the use of a conceptual balance ledger between family members offer helpful tools for building family communication.

MEDICATION COMPLIANCE AND THE IMPORTANCE OF COMMUNICATING WITH PHYSICIANS. Margaret's bipolar disorder was complicated by paranoid thinking and lack of insight even when on medication. Clients with bipolar disorders may exhibit a wide range of symptoms and behaviors, including mixed symptoms of mania and depression concurrently, from more to less extreme. Many will not evidence psychotic thought patterns, such as paranoia and delusions. Further, insight is usually present when clients are well regulated on medication.

As this case example emphasizes, medication noncompliance presents a particular risk of symptom relapse for clients with bipolar disorder. In Margaret's case, she not only believed she was well but held the delusion that the medication was poisonous. Consider that her agreeing to take it was in part a measure of her motivation to have more personal freedom than she could have if she remained in the hospital. While noncompliance is an issue for anyone taking medication on an ongoing basis, clients often dislike giving up the energized aspects of being manic. Another reason for noncompliance with many medications is troublesome side effects, such as Margaret's gaining weight when taking lithium. Helping clients and family understand what medications actually do, why the drug is important, what information to report to a doctor, and how to help ameliorate side effects cannot be accomplished in a few sessions. If you realize that clients are not complying or are bothered by some medication side effects, explore their concerns and then help them prepare to talk things out with their physicians. If this appears insufficient, seek written client consent to communicate with the physician yourself.

CONCLUSION. Margaret's story illustrates, in part, what medications can and cannot do. Mood stabilizers, such as lithium, Tegretol (carbamazepine), and Depakote (divalproex sodium) can help normalize mood, reducing the crippling highs of mania, and, in the case of lithium, may limit depressive symptoms. But they cannot help a client adjust to a changed sense of identity that comes with mood normalization in a person who has adjusted, if poorly, to having a mood disorder. They cannot help clients deal with complex life circumstances that may have had triggering effects on their illness. And they cannot help a client catch up developmentally when their illness has existed long enough to interrupt normal developmental tasks. Further, and this was not the case with Margaret, many clients with mental illnesses also experience some level of substance abuse or dependence. Medication in-and-of-itself will not help clients deal with their addictive or abusive use of drugs. Clients may be greatly helped in dealing with these various issues through appropriate treatment modalities (e.g., family, individual, group, chemical dependence). Margaret was able to participate actively in family therapy despite lacking insight into her illness, though insight would have increased her potential gains in therapy.

Antipsychotics, such as Risperdal, are used not just for clients with disorders in the schizophrenia spectrum but also for clients with psychotic symptoms, which sometimes occur as part of mood, anxiety, and personality disorders. For Margaret, Risperdal decreased paranoia and reduced the intensity of delusional thinking, which, in turn, increased her ability to resist her delusional thinking. Unfortunately, neither medication enabled Margaret to gain much insight into her mental illness. Margaret will need close supervision of her medication compliance. Initially, even though she was allowed to return home with her parents, it will become increasingly important for Margaret to establish an independent living situation, even though she may choose to live close to her parents. At that point, outside supervision, whether visits from her parents or a case manager, will be important to Margaret's stability as she attempts to return to school or find productive work.

Often, case management and goal-directed therapy help clients with serious mental illnesses reintegrate into the community and explore ways to be productive, whether by working for pay, volunteering, or returning to school. Clients' stability and decreased risk of relapse are greatly affected by medication compliance, family and social support, engaging in productive work, and premorbid functioning.

REFERRAL

Manic clients or depressed clients having had a manic episode should be referred to a physician for psychiatric evaluation. Clients who appear cyclothymic but who are subclinical should be monitored closely. It is unfortunate that when clients move into a hypomanic phase—or beyond it—it is often very difficult to get them into treatment because of their overwhelming feelings of well-being and power. Many clients in a severe manic phase must be mandated into a safe treatment setting. The counselor should be aware of the necessary protocol for civil commitment or confinement in the event that their client becomes psychotic. Compliance or hospitalization will be facilitated if the counselor has a trusting relationship with, or at least a clear communication route to, the family or the significant other. Individual treatment for bipolar disorder should include family education and therapy whenever possible. Family members often have issues with the client that may need addressing and that have been suppressed because of the client's illness. Reasonable concerns should be addressed with the client in a supportive way, and in family therapy if possible. Family members may benefit from exploring their own and family system issues, not just the patient's problems.

COMPLIANCE

Compliance issues found in all depressions are important in bipolar affective disorder. Compliance is complicated in bipolar affective disorder (a) by the client's desire for and sometimes dependence on the pleasurable, euphoric feelings that accompany the initial stages of mania; (b) by the impulsive nature of the manic phase of the disease; and (c) by the narrow therapeutic window within which lithium is effective. Often clients are in a hypomanic or depressed state (low lithium balance) or toxic state (high lithium balance) before they recognize it. If they go into a hypomanic state, clients are likely to discontinue their medication entirely because they feel so amazingly "well." As many therapists have discovered, helping a manic client recognize that medications are necessary cannot only be very difficult but very disconcerting as well due to the client's feelings of omniscience. Compliance is also complicated among bipolar affective disorder clients who are depressed because they may be agitated, hypervigilant, or frankly paranoid about their medication. In these situations, a liaison with the client's physician is very important. Liaison with the family of origin is important as well; however, this liaison should be developed only to the extent that the family is supportive and has a successful record of helping the client monitor behavioral difficulties. Otherwise, family therapy, not liaison, is called for. Studies have shown that medication compliance occurs best when patients are on appropriate medications, which may include multiple mood stabilizers (Saklad, 1997).

PHARMACOKINETICS

Lithium, one of the basic elements of chemistry, is a positively charged ion. Neurons within the body react to lithium in a manner similar to sodium or potassium. Lithium is administered orally in a salt form and rapidly absorbed. Lithium is not protein bound, and it is not metabolized. About 95% of lithium is excreted unchanged in the urine. Passage of lithium across the blood-brain barrier (BBB) and placental barrier occurs easily and can produce teratogenic effects (developmental defects in utero) in infants. Because lithium is similar to sodium (found in table salt) in both size and electrical charge, the body's lithium level is influenced by the sodium level. Patients with high sodium levels excrete more lithium, while low sodium levels trigger the body to retain greater amounts of lithium. Thus, if clients lower their ordinary salt intake (through dieting, for example), more lithium will be retained in the body. Then, if they take in large amounts of table salt when they go off their diets, a toxic level of lithium will be reached in a very short time. Clients should have the relationship between lithium and table salt explained clearly and often. The activities that make clients' salt levels fluctuate (diet, exercise, and sweating, for example) need to be fully discussed. Lithium's half-life is dependent on kidney functioning, with the average adult lithium half-life being 24 hours (Olin et al., 1998). There are a variety of trade names for lithium; among the most common are Eskalith, Lithane, Lithium Carbonate, Lithium Citrate, Lithobid, and Lithonate.

MECHANISM AND ACTIONS

The mechanisms of action for lithium's effects on both mania and depression are not fully understood. As stated above, lithium decreases mania by stabilizing the presynaptic membrane in such a way that 5-HT and NE can be reuptaken into the terminal vesicles. How this creates antidepressive effects is less clear. However, this may be accomplished by stabilizing the postsynaptic receptors so that NE can bind in a more effective way or by effects on the endocrine system (Govoni & Hayes, 1994). Although lithium crosses the BBB quickly, the antimanic effect is delayed, usually for one to two weeks. During this delay period, antipsychotics (for example, phenothiazines such as Thorazine) may be used to control manic episodes.

LITHIUM'S SIDE EFFECTS AND TOXICITY

Lithium's side effects are dose dependent, meaning larger doses will produce more extreme adverse effects. Lithium has a narrow therapeutic window with no great difference between effective and toxic doses. To prevent toxicity, patients are monitored for the appearance of adverse physical side effects (nausea and vomiting, for example) and by careful observation of lithium blood levels (Schatzberg & Cole, 1986). It is not certain whether lithium causes kidney damage in otherwise healthy patients. However, if there is a personal or family history of kidney dysfunction, kidney function should be closely monitored. Finally, because it is teratogenic, lithium treatment should be avoided during pregnancy if at all possible. Other drugs should be substituted.

EARLY SIDE EFFECTS.   Symptoms that often precede normal adjustment to lithium treatment are nausea, fine hand tremor, **polyuria** (increased urination), and **polydipsia** (increased thirst). These side effects usually subside within several weeks and are considered to be an inconvenience rather than a disabling condition. Another noted side effect is weight gain. Unfortunately, this unwanted effect discourages medication compliance.

EARLY WARNINGS OF MILD TOXICITY.   Early warnings of toxicity include diarrhea, nausea, vomiting, sedation, lack of coordination, slurred speech, and increasing confusion. Reduction in lithium dosage is the recommended treatment in cases of mild toxicity. Severe toxicity can lead to seizures, coma, and death. Unfortunately, symptoms of toxicity are similar to early side effects. Lithium intake should be reduced and the client immediately referred back to his or her physician for consultation should there be concerns about toxic effects (Olin et al., 1998).

DOSAGE.   Lithium dosage will vary depending on the phase of the illness and the side effects experienced by the patient. In the acute manic phase, the normal dose is 600 mg three times a day or, if using a time-released drug form of lithium, 900 mg twice a day. Lithium blood levels are checked twice weekly during the acute phase. Effective lithium blood levels are usually within 1–1.5 meq/liter range. In the maintenance phase, weekly visits to the physician are recommended during the first month until the patient is stabilized. After stabilization on lithium, blood level range is 0.6–1.2 meq/liter. Lithium doses in this phase will vary but are usually 300 mg three or four times a day. Lithium levels should be monitored every two to three months (Olin et al., 1998).

Patients should be advised to take lithium immediately after meals or with food or milk to avoid stomach upset. It is also recommended that patients drink 8 to 12 glasses of water a day, maintain as salt-free a diet as possible, and avoid using diuretics, including coffee and alcohol (Olin et al., 1998). It is particularly important to note that many clients with bipolar illness have histories of self-medicating with alcohol and other substances that can enormously complicate drug treatment and psychotherapy. Therapists need to explore the client's alcohol and other drug use extensively as they assess the client's self-sufficiency.

ALTERNATE TREATMENTS FOR BIPOLAR AFFECTIVE DISORDER

Even though lithium is a first-line drug in the treatment of mania and bipolar disorder, there are other drugs coming into use as first-line agents. Approximately 20–30% of patients with bipolar affective disorder are unresponsive to or do not tolerate lithium (Maxmen, 1991). When other first-line drugs are not effective (carbamazepine, for example) and a patient cannot take lithium, the depression and mania may be treated separately. Alternate treatments for mania include antipsychotics, while antidepressants may be used for the depression (see Figures 2-1 and 2-2).

Haloperidol (Haldol) or drugs in the phenothiazine class are also used for mania and are, sometimes, more effective in the treatment of severe mania. However, the side effects of antipsychotics are more troublesome. Additionally, the concomitant use of antipsychotics and lithium may increase the chance of precipitating the potentially fatal neuroleptic malignant syndrome (see Chapter 4).

As we have indicated previously, anticonvulsants are sometimes more effective than lithium in treating rapidly cycling patients. The benzodiazepine clonazepam (Klonopin), carbamazepine (Tegretol), and valproic acid (Depakene) have all been used as alternatives to lithium therapy (Ellenor & Dishman, 1996).

CONCLUSION

The study of depression and bipolar disorder is proceeding rapidly from both etiological and treatment directions. Biochemists involved in developing and testing antidepressant and antimania drugs have helped treatment specialists provide better care; clinicians have supplied invaluable information to research and development specialists. Because combatting depression is financially rewarding, research has been hastened. However, the very success of antidepressant medications in relieving many of the symptoms—and, often, many of the underlying causal features of depression—has produced a backlash. This backlash has taken the form of media exposés of the overprescription of antidepressant medications or inadequate monitoring of long-term drug therapy. It is our hope that clients will be referred to physicians for screening for medication (a) only after an adequate regime of talk therapy has failed to provide needed relief and (b) only if long-term use of the medication is closely monitored.

CHAPTER 2 REVIEW QUESTIONS

1. Describe and differentiate exogenous from endogenous depression.
2. Define and provide support for the biological amine hypothesis of depression.
3. When treating depression, what characteristics should we consider when deciding between cognitive versus antidepressant therapies versus a combination approach?
4. List common misconceptions of treatment about depression.
5. Under what circumstances should a client be referred to a psychiatrist or family physician for evaluation of need for medication?
6. Describe important features of Jan's case and provide a list of situations that might provide the basis for a decision to reevaluate and refer a client for a medical assessment.
7. Describe the different classes of antidepressants including tricyclics, MAOI inhibitors, and SSRIs and other second generation medications for depression.
8. Why might one of these classes of drugs be used as opposed to another?
9. How does unipolar affective disorder, or depression, differ from bipolar affective disorder?
10. Discuss what may occur physiologically when a patient takes an overdose of a tricyclic antidepressant. What patients are most at risk?
11. Describe the actions and therapeutic window for lithium.
12. Describe the medication compliance concerns that may develop with bipolar clients.
13. What are the early warnings of lithium toxicity?
14. Describe alternate medication treatments for people with bipolar disorder.

WEB RESOURCES ABOUT DEPRESSION

In your Internet browser, either Netscape or Internet Explorer, there is a blank space available where you can type the following URL addresses. URL addresses are universal resource locations that start with the letters "http://," and show you a page of information on the Internet. Type any of the following URL addresses into that space and press return in order to go to that page. A variety of access buttons (highlighted words that you may point and click on) are available for further information.

Please note that because of the continuously changing sites, we cannot guarantee that pages will remain at their location address. If pages are incomplete, use the address without the last part of the extension (instead of using http://www.mentalhealth.com/fr20.html, use only http://www.mentalhealth.com).

A. http://www.mentalhealth.com/fr20.html. What information does this URL address provide?

This page lists descriptions, diagnoses, and treatment and research findings on 52 of the most common mental disorders. (Examples include depression and bipolar disorder). The 67 most common psychiatric drugs (for example, Imipramine and Prozac) including indications, warnings, adverse affects, and dosage are provided.

How can this page be used?

The left side of the screen contains a list of the most common mental disorders. To select a disorder, click on its name.

Information on each disorder includes the following:

American description   Research on diagnosis, treatment, and cause
European description   Information booklets
Treatment information   Magazine articles

The bottom of the screen contains a list of topics. To select topics about medication, diagnosis, or treatment of various disorders, click on its name. Information on medication includes the following:

Pharmacology   Indications
Contraindications Warnings
Precautions   Adverse Effects

B. http://www.ndmda.org/depover.htm
C. http://www.psycom.net/depression.central.html
D. http://depression.com/

WEB RESOURCES ABOUT BIPOLAR DISORDER

In your Internet browser, either Netscape or Internet Explorer, there is a blank space available where you can type the following URL addresses. URL addresses are universal resource locations that start with the letters "http://," and show you a page of information on the Internet. Type any of the following URL addresses into that space and press return in order to go to that page. A variety of access buttons (highlighted words that you may point and click on) are available for further information.

Please note that because of the continuously changing sites, we cannot guarantee that pages will remain at their location address. If pages are incomplete, use the address without the last part of the extension (instead of using http://www.pendulum.org/info.htm, use http://www.pendulum.org/).

A. http://www.pendulum.org/info.htm

What information does this URL address provide?

This page lists a variety of topics from several mental health resources regarding the nature, diagnosis, and treatment of bipolar disorder. For example, a brochure from the National Institute of Mental Health regarding the nature of bipolar disorder, diagnosis of bipolar disorder based on the Diagnostic and Statistical Manual of Disorders - IV, and Internet Mental Health's recommendations for treatment are provided.

How can this page be used?

On the left of the screen, categories of information are presented. To find information within a category, click on the word. For example, the "Articles" category, when pressed, makes available a page with different articles such as "Research Continues on Bipolar Disorder" and "An Update on the Search for Genes for Bipolar Disorder." Click the topic to find out information. Other categories, such as "Writings," "Medications," and "Support" are available.

On the middle of the screen, four topics, "General Information, Diagnosis, Treatment, and Miscellaneous" are boldfaced. Click on this topic to find out information about the topic. For example, upon clicking the "Treatment" topic, "The Expert Consensus Guideline Series: Treatment of Bipolar Disorder" and other perspectives are topics that, when clicked, provide detailed information.

B. http://www.mentalhealth.com/fr20.html

C. http://www.nami.org/bipolar/bipolar.html.

D. http://bipolar.cmhc.com/

3

ANXIETY AND THE ANXIOLYTICS

SLEEP DISORDERS AND THE HYPNOTICS

This chapter provides an introduction to the underlying causes of anxiety as well as to the relationship between its etiology and treatment. We also discuss the referral issues involved, such as the circumstances under which clients should be referred for screening for anxiolytics and when a client should not take anxiolytics. Later in the chapter, we cover the etiology and treatment of panic attacks. Finally, we discuss various sleep disorders and recommended treatments, including the use of hypnotic agents to treat some of these disorders.

ANXIETY

Psychology, from its earliest psychodynamic beginnings to modern existentialism, has viewed anxiety as the central dilemma of social existence. It is not surprising, therefore, that social anxiety is the most common psychological problem or that anxiety is the central concern of psychotherapy. Neither, then, should it be surprising that antianxiety drugs, also referred to as **anxiolytics** or **minor tranquilizers**, are the most widely used psychiatric medications. Seventy percent of all psychiatric medications prescribed are anxiolytics, and the majority of those are sedative-hypnotic benzodiazepines (BZDs). The high prescription rate for antianxiety agents (70% of which are prescribed for women) is probably not explained by reference to any single cause. Contributing factors are the high levels of stress under which individuals (particularly women) live and work and the continued "medicalization" of anxiety. Over 65 million prescriptions for BZD medications are written each year (Garvey, 1990). This is a staggering number given that anxiety is normal and necessary to protect us from risky or foolish behavior, that BZDs produce both physical and psychological dependence and are widely abused, and that BZDs are potentially fatal when taken in amounts far above recommended doses or are combined with alcohol or other system-depressing drugs that commonly produce additive or supra-additive effects.

When anxiolytics are prescribed without an adequate psychological assessment, the patient is put at risk in several ways. First, deeper personality problems underlying the anxious feelings may be further suppressed. At the same time, because BZDs loosen impulse control, underlying hostilities toward self or others may rise to the surface and be acted on explosively. For example, anxiety often masks depression. Depression coupled with low impulse control accounts for a majority of suicides. Second, because BZDs and barbiturates are dependency-producing or addicting, there is disagreement about whether they should be taken prophylactically for long periods of time. Third, physicians who are not in the mainstream of psychiatric services but who prescribe BZDs may not encourage patients to begin anxiety management psychotherapy (AMP) in a timely way or at all. Fourth, like all sedative **hypnotics**, BZDs can loosen impulse control; patients without adequate drug education and adequate self-monitoring may impulsively take risks (take drugs they would ordinarily be too anxious to take, for example).

BZDs need careful controls (Tyrer & Seivewright, 1984). In our view (a view shared by many in the drug treatment field), BZDs should rarely be used for more than several weeks. Long-term BZD therapy should be considered only in the event that psychotherapy has clearly been shown to be unsuccessful.

DIAGNOSIS

The DSM-IV (APA, 1994) describes a wide range of anxiety disorders, including generalized anxiety disorder, simple phobia, social phobia, obsessive-compulsive disorder, post-traumatic stress disorder, panic disorders, and agoraphobia without history of panic disorders. All anxiety disorders commonly include motor tension, autonomic hyperactivity (shortness of breath, palpitations, sweating, dizziness), vigilance, and scanning. Each specific disorder includes further characteristic features. Individuals with anxiety disorders are often successful at controlling their anxiety by avoiding situations that trigger it or by self-medication with alcohol. Avoidance may lead to a constriction of interpersonal and economic circumstances. For example, people with social phobias may not be able to advance in their jobs if advancement requires making speeches, teaching, or giving presentations.

Many anxious people medicate their problems with alcohol even though alcohol, because of rebound hyperexcitability, may exacerbate those problems. Unfortunately, like the other sedative-hypnotic drugs, alcohol can produce dependence and, for many, addiction.

Anxiety disorders may be divided into those that are spontaneous and thought to arise from genetic predisposition (generalized anxiety and obsessive-compulsive disorders, for example), those that arise through a conditioning experience (post-traumatic stress disorder (PTSD), for example), and signal anxieties that are thought to arise from unconscious conflicts. Each of these disorders can give rise to or be accompanied by panic attacks.

ETIOLOGY

Arousal elements in both normal and abnormal anxiety are caused by either a decrease of an inhibitory neurotransmitter (GABA, for example) or an overabundance of an excitatory neurotransmitter (norepinephrine, for example) or both. Interpretation of an arousal state as anxiety, however, is dependent upon or mediated by culture-bound cognitions. Thus, what is happy excitement for one person may be anxiety for another, even though the physiological states are not distinguishably different. Very low levels of inhibitory neurotransmitters and very high levels of excitatory neurotransmitters are known to cause strokes, seizures, paranoia, and panic. Thus, abrupt discontinuation of a tranquilizing medication (inhibitory, sedative-hypnotic BZD, for example) and the subsequent rapid rise of excitation can cause the same symptoms as an overdose of a stimulant medication (adrenaline, for example). This state is called **rebound hyperexcitability**.

Panic states are caused by extreme reactivity of the centers in the brain that ordinarily alert the individual to impending danger. These centers, comprising the ascending reticular activating system (ARAS) of the brain, are rich in norepinephrine (NE). In the panic condition, these centers are bathed in NE, and the level of inhibitory neurotransmitter (GABA and serotonin or 5-HT, for example) is insufficient to quiet the system (Julien, 1996).

Further, in areas of the brain concerned with sleep, feeding, and sexual activity, 5-HT acts as an inhibitory neurotransmitter in opponent process with the excitatory neurotransmitter NE. Opponent process in this context implies acting in opposition to the excitatory effects exerted by NE. Thus, raising levels of 5-HT, as most second generation antidepressants do, down-regulates activity in these areas. Heterocyclic drugs known to raise 5-HT are fluoxetine (Prozac), sertraline (Zoloft), and fluvoxamine (Luvox). Both fluoxetine and sertraline also down-regulate sensitivity of NE receptors, which accounts for their ability to decrease depression without increasing mania as the tricyclics often do. One tricyclic antidepressant, clomipramine (Anafranil), is also thought to specifically raise levels of serotonin and is successfully used in treating obsessive-compulsive disorder, which appears related to abnormally low levels of serotonin.

Of particular importance is the regulation of proper levels of 5-HT in the brain's pontine raphe nuclei, a group of nerve cells that serves as a filtering system for incoming stimuli. 5-HT filters the flood of incoming information, letting through the most important and filtering out the less relevant. Interestingly, when **lysergic acid diethylamide (LSD)** competes with 5-HT at serotonin-2 receptors, it allows an unfiltered flood of sensory data that overloads the system and causes a wide range of cognitive and emotional distortions (Julien, 1996). These include, but are not limited to, feelings of unreality; novel cognitions, perceptions, and emotions; disorientation to time; and depersonalization or hyperpersonalization. Further, many users experience sleeplessness, anxiety, paranoia, and panic. These last characteristics are caused by inadequate levels of serotonin (5-HT).

Confirmation of the inhibitory and regulatory functions of serotonin, and therefore the utility of the serotonin reuptake blocking antianxiety medications, comes from several divergent sources. Unfortunately, this picture is complicated by several factors. First, the final action of serotonin is not an inhibitory one in all areas of the brain. If serotonin acts to inhibit an area of the limbic system whose function is to suppress an emotion or behavior, serotonin can be said to activate that emotion. Thus, 5-HT can act as an antidepressant in its final outcome, especially in its effects on depression through regulation of the sleep cycle. A major part of the utility of fluoxetine in lowering depression may well be in its regulation of sleep. Second, and less well understood, most neurotransmitters can be either excitatory or inhibitory depending on where their effects are measured. What is clearly inhibitory in one locus of the brain may well be excitatory in another.

In conclusion, we are discovering that low serotonin is responsible for a wide range of emotional disturbances that includes both depression and anxiety. Therefore, use of medications that enhance 5-HT is likely to rise. At present, 800,000 prescriptions are being written each month for Prozac alone. Zoloft, another heterocyclic antidepressant, is also rapidly gaining hold in the marketplace. Because it has fewer side effects and drug interactions and has rapid onset, Zoloft is often prescribed for geriatric depression and agitation.

TREATMENT

Anxiety is often lifelong unless treated because the predisposition to anxiety is genetically driven. Children with a first-degree family member suffering from anxiety will also suffer anxiety in approximately 50% of cases—even when they are not raised by their biological parents (Barlow, 1988). Second, learned anxiety generalizes. When anxiety is conditioned through a particular event (punishment, for example), the site of punishment and other conditions surrounding the punishment may be sufficient to evoke the anxiety over an extended period of time. Third, anticipation of panic is itself a potent causal agent of further anxiety. Fear reactions may be so aversive in and of themselves that anticipation of that fear may give rise to anticipatory anxiety that spirals upward in intensity. This anticipation is usually pushed forward by visualization of oneself in the panic condition. Fourth, unresolved psychological problems can produce anxiety.

Signal anxieties appear to arise from unconscious conflicts. In these cases, anxiety results from the activity of holding painful memories (sexual abuse, for example) under repression. From a psychodynamic perspective, the anxiety will only dissipate when these underlying issues have surfaced and been worked through. Our experience indicates that anxiety management programs that include progressive relaxation, desensitization through reciprocal inhibition, and cognitive restructuring are not usually successful over the long run with individuals whose anxiety stems from deeper, unresolved issues.

The prognosis for controlling anxiety through a combination of anxiolytics and psychotherapy is best if panic attacks, obsessive-compulsive features, major depressive episodes, and simple phobias are not central features of the condition. Stress-related and generalized anxieties have the best prognosis and yield to drug treatment in about 65% of cases without psychotherapy (Barlow & Cerny, 1988). Presumably, this rate would increase substantially when drugs and psychotherapy are utilized together.

Psychotherapy, primarily anxiety management programs (AMP), should be used in place of drug therapy wherever feasible for a number of reasons. First, because antianxiety medications are often addicting, they should not be taken for extended periods (e.g., more than two weeks). Second, psychotherapy is useful in identifying and de-escalating anticipatory anxiety preparatory to panic incidents. Third, psychotherapy is less expensive over the long run and can support lifestyle changes that will reduce many of the health deficits that arise from anxiety and stress. And fourth, evaluation and treatment of underlying problems that may decrease drug treatment should be ongoing. See Box 3-1 for suggested uses of AMP and drug treatment.

Although anxiety about medication is common, it can be a significant treatment barrier for clients with anxiety disorders. Verbalizations of fear about the medication are frequent. Even if a client has no experience with the prescribed medication, clients often provide numerous reasons supporting their avoidance of drug therapy. Therapists need to educate fearful clients on the benefits of medication and encourage them to be compliant with their physician's advice. The case of C illustrates this point.

CASE STUDY: OBSESSIVE COMPULSIVE ANXIETY DISORDER

Cheryl was a 22-year-old female. An only child, Cheryl chose to live with her parents because she felt they needed her presence. Assessment revealed that Cheryl's father was disabled by severe OCD and depression, but he took medication only for the depression. Cheryl explained that four years ago he had a bad reaction to Anafranil (an antidepressant used to treat OCD). Cheryl also suffered from severe symptoms of OCD. In her initial session, she described how she spent most of her time decorating and redecorating her bedroom. She

---

Box 3-1   Anxiety Management Programs and Drug Treatment

Drug treatment without a formal anxiety management program is indicated if
- stressors leading to episodic anxiety are found to be of short duration and are situation limited,
- relaxation or other techniques are sufficient to trigger high levels of anxiety or panic episodes, or
- client has a history of lack of progress with at least two psychotherapy techniques, one of which is a structured anxiety management program.

AMP alone should be considered if
- client fails to respond to adequate trials of two anxiolytics or has an inability to tolerate medication side effects,
- client has only a partial response to adequate doses of anxiolytics,
- client fails or exhibits only a partial response to other less structured psychotherapeutic methods,
- stress or environmental triggers predominate, or
- cognitions are the most salient triggers of anxiety.

In addition, the following conditions should be met when using AMP alone:
- The client has no previous diagnosis of untreated affective (depressive) disorder.
- Panic attacks occur no more than once a year.
- Anxiety is not accompanied by mania or hypomania.
- The client is not presently dependent on or abusing alcohol or other drugs.

Sources: Barlow, 1988; Barlow & Cerny, 1988; Beck & Emery, 1985.

---

had painted her room six times in the last four months and was still dissatisfied with the color. Also, she indicated that anything she did had to be done at least twice. Cheryl related that her obsessive thoughts and compulsive behaviors were very intrusive not only for her but also for her whole family. Although she was reluctant to see a psychiatrist, with support she finally agreed. The psychiatrist diagnosed her with severe OCD and prescribed Anafranil, but she refused the medication, citing her father's prior negative experience. Because Prozac had been successful in reducing symptoms of OCD, she agreed to give Prozac a try. Unfortunately, Cheryl discontinued it after seven weeks because she heard on a news broadcast that Prozac might have caused bizarre behavior in some clients.

At times, Cheryl's symptoms became so severe that it prevented her from sleeping and attending her counseling sessions. Cheryl's therapist continued to try to educate her about cognitive behavioral strategies, about the biological basis of OCD, and about the possible benefits of medication. After much encouragement from her therapist and in consultation with her physician, Cheryl agreed to try Luvox (fluvoxamine) for symptoms of OCD and Klonopin (clonazepam) for sleep. When Cheryl stayed on her medication, her symptoms were manageable. Unfortunately, however, whenever she became fearful and obsessed on the possible negative effects of her prescriptions (a common feature of clients with OCD), she discontinued them without consulting her doctor, family, or therapist, and the disabling symptoms of OCD would reappear.

Cheryl's case clearly illustrates how the symptoms (obsessive thoughts and generalized anxiety) can prevent a client from complying with recommended treatment. Therapists must be patient, persistent, and creative in trying to help clients with the entire range of their anxiety disorder. Because it is necessary to present the same information numerous times, creativity in presenting the educational materials and stamina in working through a tested anxiety management program are very important. Also, because working with anxious clients can be frustrating for therapists, a nonjudgmental understanding and acceptance of the underlying features of clients' resistance is critical.

TREATMENT CONSIDERATIONS: THE CLIENT'S POINT OF VIEW

Individuals presenting for treatment of anxiety have often moved through a wide variety of precipitating events. Anxiety is often produced by both legal and illegal drugs, including the sedative hypnotics prescribed to help solve the anxiety problem in the first place. For many people, ordinary behaviors (speaking to a group of people, for example) may be interpreted as frightening, even though there is no clear threat. In these cases, the anticipatory anxiety becomes painful and embarrassing. Further, many activities thought necessary to survive in the modern world are, by the very nature of human evolutionary history, stressful. Human beings are not well designed for jobs that require constant vigilance or high levels of autonomic stimulation like those of air traffic controllers or long-distance pilots. Finally, people who take stimulant drugs (cocaine, amphetamines, and especially large amounts of coffee) often experience debilitating panic attacks. Stimulant abusers who are having panic attacks often present themselves for treatment or referral to get prescriptions for tranquilizers so they can continue their drug abuse with less anxiety. Furthermore, a wide range of physical problems can cause anxiety, irritability, and agitation. Box 3-2 lists some of the more common conditions associated with panic and anxiety symptoms.

Most people discover at one time or another that alcohol is a powerful sedative hypnotic and anxiolytic, even if it is effective only over the short run. Unfortunately, like the majority of anxiolytic sedative hypnotics (benzodiazepines, for example), alcohol can be addictive and often causes rebound hyperexcitability when it is abruptly discontinued. Hyperexcitability due to abrupt discontinuation of long-term use of sedative hypnotics can cause strokes, seizures, feelings of depersonalization, anxiety, and panic attacks. Long-term withdrawal symptoms (in many cases, longer than one year) make treatment more difficult and almost impossible if these effects are not taken into consideration and dealt with in therapy.

Box 3-2   Organic Conditions Associated with Panic and Anxiety Symptoms

- Asthmatic conditions
- Audiovestibular system disturbance
- Cardiac arrhythmias
- Cushing syndrome (increased cortisol output)
- Hyperthyroidism (excessive thyroid activity)
- Hyperventilation
- Hypoglycemia (low blood sugar)
- Hypoparathyroidism (deficient parathyroid activity)
- Mitral valve prolapse
- Pheochromocytoma (adrenal tumor)
- Postconcussion syndromes
- Temporal lobe epilepsy

Source: Szeinbach & Summers, 1992.

Long-term withdrawal symptoms include irritability, depression, drug craving, mood swings, and an exacerbation of the anxiety that the drugs were originally prescribed to control. When either alcohol or the BZDs are being abused for their euphoric effects, tolerance develops so that a higher and higher dose must be taken to produce the same effect. However, some studies have found that individuals without a history of alcohol or drug abuse who are prescribed BZDs usually do not increase their reported dose (Garvey, 1990; Roy-Byrne, 1992). Individuals who routinely use alcohol or short-acting BZDs are likely to go through *daily* rebound hyperexcitability.

Given these problems, the difficult withdrawal from prescription sedative hypnotics and the high relapse back to BZDs for anxiety sufferers (Roy-Byrne, 1992), many counselors in the drug treatment field believe that these medications cause more problems than they cure.

THE THERAPIST'S POINT OF VIEW: THE MEDICATED CLIENT

Counselors are faced with several central concerns in treating anxious clients who are being medicated. First, there is evidence that having a client on an anxiolytic interferes with anxiety management programs (AMP) by temporarily interrupting the connection between the stimulus (e.g., thoughts of speaking in public) and the response (anxiety) so that desensitization learning cannot occur (Sanderson & Wetzler, 1993). If no anxiety exists in the medicated client, no graded series of cognitive-emotional exercises to diminish the stress can take place. Reciprocal inhibition techniques do not work if there is no low-level stress to be inhibited; again, no learning takes place. Second, anxiety that arises from depression and that is treated with anxiolytics may exacerbate

depression and put some clients at higher risk for suicide. This is true because anxiolytics are depressants on the one hand while their anxiolytic properties weaken impulse control on the other. Approximately 60% of all suicides are committed by depressed individuals under the influence of sedative-hypnotic drugs, usually alcohol (Julien, 1996).

Fortunately, unlike the barbiturate drugs, a dose of BZDs 60 times larger than a normal therapeutic dose is usually required for an adult male to commit suicide, assuming no other sedative hypnotic, including alcohol, has been consumed. Even in cases of large doses ingested, patients have rarely been successful in their attempts because suppression of breathing by BZDs is a lengthy and reversible process. However, alcohol and other depressants potentiate or geometrically increase the effects of the BZDs so that fewer are needed for suicide. Anxious patients who are also depressed should not be prescribed either barbiturates or synthetic barbiturates (methaqualone, glutethimide, or meprobamate), which are all life threatening at less than 20 times the usual dose necessary to relieve anxiety or sleeplessness (Lickey & Gordon, 1995).

Anxiety management approaches are often sabotaged by clients dependent on sedative-hypnotic drugs because clients believe the drugs are crucial to their well-being. The AMP tries to wean clients away from their drugs, and, thus, client and program objectives are headed in opposite directions. To win, the client has only to discontinue treatment. A strong therapeutic alliance with the client and the client's physician is crucial for AMP to be effective. Often, alcohol or drug treatment is necessary before long-term sedativists can profit from AMP. Clients who are suspected of being dependent on sedative hypnotics, especially alcohol, should not be advised to discontinue their use abruptly. They need to be assessed for medical detoxification. This is especially true if the client is older or has had any symptoms of delirium tremens (DTs).

REFERRAL

Anxious clients should be referred for psychiatric screening for an anxiolytic under any of the following circumstances:

- The client is too anxious or paranoid to take advantage of a cognitive-behavioral anxiety management program.
- AMP or at least one other form of psychotherapy has been shown to be ineffective for this client at this time.
- There is a history of a first-degree family member whose similar anxiety responds favorably to anxiolytics and who has not formed a drug dependency.

AMP should be initiated in conjunction with the drug therapy as soon as the client's anxiety has been reduced to a level that makes AMP possible.

Barlow and Cerny (1988) and others (Barlow, 1988; Beck & Emery, 1985) have suggested that clients should be referred for psychiatric screening for both medical and psychiatric conditions under any of the following circumstances:

- Client has a history or family history of depression, including bipolar disorder.
- Client has a history or family history of psychosis.
- Client has a history or family history of endocrine or hormonal problems.
- Client has a history of brain injury or life-threatening injury.
- Client has a history of impulsive behavior, including life-threatening behavior.

Clients should not take anxiolytics, especially barbiturates and benzodiazepines, if they

- are not willing to consider psychotherapy as a co-therapy
- are drinkers or illicit drug users
- are using anxiolytics for more than three evenings in a row as a sleep medication (tolerance for their sleep-inducing effects develops quickly)
- have used anxiolytics for more than two months without a drug holiday lasting several weeks
- are increasing their dosage beyond the ordinary range for nontolerant persons
- are keeping large numbers of pills on hand, or
- are getting refills without consulting a physician

ANTIANXIETY AGENTS

Antianxiety agents are more effective in anticipatory situations than in panic conditions. To avoid the lifelong use of antianxiety drugs, the source of the anxiety must be investigated and eliminated. Psychotherapy should be adjunct treatment for anxiety.

Other terms used to describe this collection of drugs are *minor tranquilizers* or *anxiolytics*. The term *minor tranquilizer* implies similarities to a group of drugs called *major tranquilizers* (antipsychotics); however, they are not the same. Use of the word *minor* to describe this group of addictive anxiolytics was a marketing strategy by the drug companies to smooth their introduction into the marketplace, a tactic that has had enormous success. BZDs are an example of a popular class of minor tranquilizer; phenothiazines are an example of a class of major tranquilizers. Table 3-1 provides a comparison of the major actions for both groups of drugs and illustrates the differences.

Therapeutic Effects of Minor Tranquilizers: The onset of the desired effects of a minor tranquilizer can occur quickly, in anywhere from 10 minutes to several

Table 3-1   A Comparison of the Effects of Major and Minor Tranquilizers

Minor Tranquilizers (Benzodiazepines or BZDs)	*Major Tranquilizers (phenothiazines)*
Sedation	Sedation
Antianxiety	Extrapyramidal side effects
Central muscle relaxers	Neuroleptic state:
	Psychomotor slowing
	Emotional quieting (fewer
	hallucinations and delusions)
	Affective indifference
High addiction potential	No addiction potential

Source: Julien, 1998.

hours, because BZDs are rapidly absorbed into the bloodstream (Ponterotto, 1985).

Dangers of Minor Tranquilizers: Tolerance, causing an increase in dosage, psychological dependence and addiction, and the potential to produce fetal abnormalities (Maxmen, 1991).

Side Effects of Minor Tranquilizers: Drowsiness, ataxia (lack of coordination) with high doses, slurred speech, and other signs of CNS depression are common side effects associated with antianxiety agents. Potential for successful suicide is moderate to low unless this medication is used with other CNS depressants (Szeinbach & Summers, 1992).

Precautions: Abrupt discontinuation of antianxiety agents that have been used for a long time is ill advised (Swonger & Matejski, 1991). Rebound hyperactivity may produce strokes, seizures, and panic states. This class of drugs should not be used for primary depression, primary psychosis (they may worsen psychotic agitation), or personality disorders (Olin et al., 1998). Again, due to their disinhibiting properties, BZDs should not be used in depressed clients because it may lead to an increased risk of suicide. Also, extreme caution should be taken in prescribing antianxiety agents to a client with a history of dependence on sedatives or alcohol (Wright, 1996).

BENZODIAZEPINE ANTIANXIETY AGENTS

BZDs are often the treatment of choice for anxiety. BZDs do not cure anxiety but do reduce symptoms. Removal of all symptoms may not be desirable because anxiety is considered both an emotion and an essential drive and is primarily connected to choice and uncertainty, both of which are necessary for functioning in the modern world (Leccese, 1991). Table 3-2 lists antianxiety drugs and their most common uses.

Table 3-2   Specific Antianxiety Benzodiazepines and Their Uses

Trade Name	Generic Name	Daily Doses (Divided into 2–4 Doses)	Elimination Half-Life in Hours (Range)	Uses
Ativan	lorazepam	1–10 mg	10–24	Anxiety associated with depression; preanesthetic sedative; acute mania; lithium-resistant bipolar disorder
Centrax	praxepam	20–40 mg	50–100	Short-term for anxiety
Klonipin	clonazepam	.25–1.5 mg	18–50	Panic attacks; certain types of seizures; acute mania; lithium-resistant bipolar disorder
Dalmane	flurazepam	15–30 mg*	70–160	Primarily for sleep
Dormalin, Doral	quazepam	7.5–15 mg*	25–50	Primarily for sleep
Halcion	triazolam	.125–0.5 mg*	1.5–5	Primarily for sleep
Librium	chlordiazepoxide	15–300 mg	8–24	Preoperative anxiety (given a few days before surgery); acute alcohol withdrawal
Paxipam	halazepam	20–160 mg	10–20**	Acute anxiety and sedation
Prosom	estazolam	1–2 mg*	13–35	Primarily for sleep
Restoril	temazepam	15–30 mg*	8–35	Primarily for sleep
Serax	oxazepam	30–120 mg	5–15	Anxiety associated with depression
Tranxene	chlorazepate	15–60 mg	50–100	Adjunct to seizure treatment; acute alcohol withdrawal; certain types of seizures
Valium	diazepam	2–40 mg	20–50	Acute alcohol withdrawal; adjunct muscle relaxer; adjunct anticonvulsant and preoperative; unlabeled use—panic attacks
Versed	midazolam	—	1.5–4.5	Preoperative sedation; sedation before and during selected medical procedures
Xanax	alprazolam	0.5–1.5 mg	11–18	Panic disorder; unlabeled use—agoraphobia with social phobia; premenstrual syndrome

*One dose daily taken at bedtime
**Second active compound in blood, Nordiazepam, elimination half-life of 50–100 hours
***Injectable form only

Sources: Nursing99 Books, 1999; Julien, 1998; Olin et al., 1998.

MISCELLANEOUS ANTIANXIETY AGENTS

Table 3-3 lists antianxiety agents other than BZDs and includes daily dosages and the most common uses for each of these agents. Table 3-4 lists antidepressants used to treat OCD.

Buspar (buspirone) is a frequently used antianxiety agent that is chemically and pharmacologically unrelated to BZDs or other sedatives or anxiolytics. Like many other effective medications, its mechanism of action is unclear. Buspar has an advantage over other drugs in that it is less sedating, has a low potential for abuse, and has no known withdrawal effects. Because it is less sedating, it is particularly beneficial for use among the elderly. However, Buspar has a slow onset of action. Buspar's side effects include dizziness, nausea, headaches, and lightheadedness (Wright, 1996). Patients taking Buspar should avoid alcohol consumption.

Table 3-3   Antianxiety Agents Other than BZD

Trade Name	Generic Name	Daily Doses (Divided into 2–4 Doses)	Uses
Adapin, Sinequan	Doxepin[1]	25–400 mg	Anxiety; depression; somatic symptoms and concerns; insomnia; guilt; lack of energy; fear; apprehension; worry
Atarax, Vistaril	Hydroxyzine (antihistamine)		Itching; preanesthesia sedative; IM for acutely disturbed or hysterical patient or for withdrawal symptoms; as adjunctive medication to permit a reduction in dosages of narcotics
BuSpar[2]	Buspirone	15–30 mg	Unlabeled use—premenstrual syndrome; anxiolytic follow up after discontinuation of BZD or alcohol consumption
Equanil, Miltown	Meprobamate[3]	800–2400 mg	Similar to barbiturates; now used rarely for sleep and anxiety

[1]Doxepin is a tricyclic antidepressant with antianxiety action.
[2]BuSpar's mechanism of action is that of a selective (serotonin) 5-HT (1A) subreceptor agonist. Like other 5-HT agonists, BuSpar also has antidepressant effects. It has not been found effective in panic situations. BuSpar is less sedating than BZDs, but CNS effects may not be as predictable. No cross-tolerance with other CNS depressants (for example, BZDs or alcohol) appear to develop. Patients taking BuSpar do not develop drug dependency; therefore, it is safer than the BZDs. Optimum results are seen in three to four weeks.
[3]Has the highest suicide and addiction risk.

Sources: Maxmen, 1991; Napoliello & Domantay, 1991; Olin et al., 1993.

Table 3-4   Antidepressants Used to Treat OCD

Trade Name	Generic Name
Anafranil	clomipramine
Luvox	fluvoximine
Paxil	paroxetine
Prozac	fluoxetine
Zoloft	sertraline

Source: Olin et al., 1998.

PANIC ATTACKS

A panic attack is a sudden episode of inappropriate intense fear, apprehension, or terror with multiple physiological symptoms. Although only around 6% of the population experience multiple panic attacks yearly (Dugas, 1987), perhaps 34% of the normal population experience one panic attack yearly (Barlow & Cerny, 1988). Thus, panic or anxiety attacks are very common. Their onset usually occurs in the late teens or mid-20s, and there is evidence of a genetic component for this disorder (Dugas, 1987).

ETIOLOGY

Spontaneous panic attacks (meaning no precipitating factor can be identified or the attacks are both uncued and unexpected) are thought to have an organic basis. A neurochemical defect is suspected in the brain's locus ceruleus (an area of the brain stem). The locus ceruleus either amplifies or dampens incoming brain messages. In a panic attack, the incoming signal is misinterpreted or overinterpreted by the locus ceruleus, relaying panic messages to other areas of the brain (Charney, Heninger, & Breier, 1984).

Panic attacks can lead to agoraphobia. An individual having panic attacks may identify many causes for these unwanted episodes, creating anticipatory anxiety. Anticipatory anxiety can lead to extreme avoidance. The culmination of this avoidance may lead to an individual refusing to leave home. With this progression in mind, agoraphobia may be considered to be a more severe variant of panic disorder (Noyes et al., 1986).

TREATMENT

Unfortunately, the most common mode of intervention for all anxiety problems is self-medication with alcohol. However, this intervention is inappropriate because alcohol use can cause rebound panic attacks. Alcohol may worsen panic attacks because even mild alcohol withdrawal will intensify the problem (Woolf, 1983). In treating panic attacks, Dugas (1987) targets three groups of symptoms:

- *emotional symptoms*, such as overwhelming fear or apprehension, fear of dying or going crazy
- *physiological signs*, such as difficult breathing, increased heart rate, dizziness, or nausea
- *anticipatory anxiety*, which leads to more avoidance

Past research has shown that antianxiety agents do a poor job of eradicating panic attacks. This is true for a combination of reasons but primarily because a dose of BZDs capable of preventing uncued and unexpected panic attacks is high enough to cause major side effects. Further, most uncued panic attacks, those not tied to specific external stimuli, occur before even the fast-acting BZDs can take effect. Cued and expected panic attacks, those caused by public speaking, for example, can be medicated successfully with a combination of a short-acting BZD and propranolol (Inderal), a beta-adrenergic blocker often prescribed to lower blood pressure, which helps control the rapid heartbeat and other physiological symptoms of norepinephrine-cued distress. Propranolol has been found to be effective in decreasing the cardiorespiratory symptoms of panic attacks while having no abuse potential.

In some cases, the emotional symptoms and physiological signs are helped by using the tricyclic antidepressant imipramine (Tofranil) at 150–200 mg daily, or clomipramine (Anafranil), a serotonin reuptake inhibitor. Monoamine oxidase inhibitor (MAOI) antidepressants, such as phenelzine (Nardil), are also used but require dietary restrictions. The second generation antidepressant Prozac (fluoxetine) has also been found to have an inhibiting effect on both anxiety and panic and, particularly, on the anxiety dimensions of obsessive-compulsive disorder. Benzodiazepines (BZDs) often complement the effects of the antidepressants in treating panic attacks by helping to alleviate the anticipatory anxiety. One BZD, Xanax (alprazolam) at a dose of at least 4 mg daily is needed for successful treatment for the associated anxiety. However, as we have indicated, chronic use of BZDs carries the risk of tolerance and dependence (Dugas, 1987; Roy-Byrne, 1992; Swonger & Matejski, 1991).

SLEEP DISORDERS

Sleep is a cyclic phenomenon. The various stages from wakefulness to deep sleep are recorded polygraphically with the assistance of an **electroencephalogram (EEG)**, which measures brain waves (Moorcroft, 1989). The five stages are beta (awake and active), alpha (relaxed and sleepy), theta (asleep), delta (very deep sleep), and **rapid eye movement (REM) sleep**, during which the body is partially paralyzed and most dreaming occurs. Paradoxically, REM sleep is autonomically closest to wakefulness, and during the night we usually move through cycles of delta and REM sleep. Each sleep stage is characterized by different brain wave patterns. Sleep stages 1 through 4 are collectively referred to as *nonrapid eye movement* (non-REM). Some of stage 3 and most of stage 4 contains delta (slow) waves. **Delta waves** represent deep, restorative sleep. The brain's neurotransmitter serotonin plays an active role in non-REM sleep, and the neurotransmitter norepinephrine is vital to REM sleep and wakeful activity. REM sleep is characterized by regular fast eye movements, muscle paralysis, and dream activity. As the night progresses, REM sleep stages increase in length and become more intense psychologically and physiologically (Riley, 1985). As people age, sleep naturally becomes shallower and shorter. Conditions in the elderly that interrupt sleep patterns are pain, frequent awakenings to urinate, cardiovascular and metabolic disorders, and overmedication (Grinspoon, 1994).

SLEEP DEPRIVATION

After a period of REM sleep deprivation, an individual will rebound by spending more sleep time in the REM stage. Effects of sleep deprivation are feelings of intense sleepiness, depressed mood, increased aggression, difficulty in maintaining prolonged concentration, perceptual distortions and, sometimes, mild hallucinations (Morris, Williams, & Lubin, 1960; Parkes, 1985). The DSM-IV categorizes sleep disorders into two main groups:

- **parasomnias**—an abnormal event during sleep
- **dyssomnias**—complaints of amount, quality, or timing of sleep (APA, 1994)

It is important to determine if the sleep problem is a sleep disorder or sleep disturbances that are frequently seen in depressive illnesses.

SLEEP DISORDERS AND RECOMMENDED TREATMENTS

Primary causes of insomnia include pain, full bladder, prostate problems, alcohol and drugs that may contain caffeine, medication side effects, irritable bowel syndrome, heart problems, infections, cancer, endocrinological and metabolic problems (especially fibromyalgia and myofascial pain syndromes), fever, acid reflux, sleep apnea, restless leg syndrome, and chronic obstructive pulmonary disease. Common psychiatric causes of sleeplessness include depression, anxiety, alcoholism and other drug addiction, mania or hypomania, schizophrenia, PTSD, and, finally, high stress.

General suggestions for improving sleep include:

- Maintain regular times to get to bed and to arise in the morning.
- Do not spend more than 8 hours in bed.
- Do not drink any drink containing caffeine (including coffee, tea, and chocolate) after noon.
- Do not drink alcohol or large amounts of any liquid before going to bed.
- Do not take naps during the day unless you suffer from chronic fatigue or narcolepsy.
- Avoid using the bed or bedroom for watching television.

- Keep the room cool and minimize noise and other distractions.
- Exercise at least 6 hours before bedtime, especially if exercise is vigorous.
- Sex before sleeping is recommended, but long-winded discussion about problems of the day is not.
- Do not stay in bed if you are not sleepy, but get up and read or do some other quiet activity; return when you feel sleepy.
- Try progressive muscle relaxation techniques.

Somnambulism (sleepwalking) is usually seen in children, who generally outgrow this sleep disorder. Approximately 10–20% of the population experience sleepwalking episodes. Sleepwalking occurs during delta wave sleep, and, contrary to popular belief, it is not the acting out of dreams. Somnambulism is more likely to occur if an individual is tired, sleep deprived, under stress, or taking sleeping pills. Recommended treatment is to protect the sleepwalker by taking specific actions such as locking doors and giving the sleepwalker a first-floor bedroom (Moorcroft, 1989).

Night terrors (sleep terror disorder or pavor nocturnus) are characterized by extreme vocalizations (usually occurring one-half to 1 hour after sleep onset), sweating, or fast heart rate (tachycardia). Night terrors are also a delta wave sleep phenomenon. Occurring mostly in children, night terrors are frequently outgrown. Benzodiazepines (BZDs), a chemical class of sedative-hypnotic drugs, suppress delta wave sleep. However, the risks associated with the use of BZDs on the developing central nervous systems of children is unknown; therefore, use of BZDs in treating night terrors is not recommended (Hauri, 1985).

Nightmares (dream anxiety disorder) differ from night terrors in that nightmares are usually associated with elaborate and frightening content. In night terrors the individual is usually unable to recall a narrative. Additionally, nightmares occur during REM sleep rather than during non-REM sleep. Recommended treatment is that parents calm and reassure their child. For adults with frequent, disturbing nightmares, psychotherapy is suggested (Wincor, 1990).

Sleep apnea (breathing-related sleep disorder) occurs mostly in men over 30 years old and is characterized by episodes of cessation in breathing, producing many "mini-arousals" throughout the night. An individual suffering from sleep apnea may not be aware of the interruptions in normal breathing. Often, the only complaints are headaches, irritability, or difficulty in daytime functioning. Two main causes for sleep apnea are (1) airway obstruction, as in enlarged tonsils, and (2) malfunctioning in the brain's respiratory centers. Treatment depends on etiology. A tonsillectomy or weight loss may eradicate the airway obstruction problem. In extreme (life-threatening) cases, a tracheostomy (airway vent in the throat) may be necessary. It is imperative to avoid all drugs with CNS depressant activity (including tranquilizers, hypnotics, sedatives, narcotics, and alcohol). Central nervous system–depressing agents are potentially lethal to an individual with sleep apnea. CNS depressants can interfere with the body's built-in mechanisms (mini-arousals) that function to block the prolonging of apnea episodes (Wincor, 1990).

Narcolepsy is characterized by uncontrolled sleep attacks of short duration. The most common features associated with narcolepsy include the following:

- excessive daytime sleepiness
- falling asleep at inopportune moments
- cataplexy, a brief episode of muscle weakness that can result from experiencing strong emotions such as laughter or anger
- sleep paralysis, an inhibition of musculature without unconsciousness (although apparently awake, the individual is unable to move)
- hypnogogic hallucinations, REM dreams that occur during wakeful sleep paralysis (APA, 1994)

However, the main symptom of narcolepsy is sleep attacks that last from 2 to 5 minutes.

Onset for narcolepsy usually occurs in adolescence, and there is evidence of a genetic basis for this disorder. Narcolepsy is thought to be caused by inappropriate neural mechanisms that produce REM sleep (Carlson, 1991). Nonpharmacologic treatment is to educate the family about narcolepsy, stressing that an individual suffering from narcolepsy is not lazy or unmotivated. Daytime naps, lasting 15 to 20 minutes, may be helpful.

CNS stimulants are used for daytime sleepiness. Because of problems with abuse and dependence when using drugs in the amphetamine class of CNS stimulants, other (often similar) types of stimulants are usually used to treat narcolepsy. Two such drugs are methylphenidate (Ritalin), which is also a frequently abused drug, and pemoline (Cylert) (Wincor, 1990).

Bruxism (teeth grinding) occurs mostly in children but is not infrequently seen among adults, especially during periods of stress. As many as 15% of children may grind their teeth while sleeping. In some children, teeth grinding is only temporary, but in others, it may be more of a problem. In some instances, a dentist is consulted for treatment. Teeth grinding has not been clearly associated with psychological problems (Moorcroft, 1989).

Insomnia is associated with a perceived decrease in the quality or quantity of sleep that affects daytime functioning. Ninety-five percent of all adults experience insomnia at least once in their lives. Diagnosis of insomnia is subjectively determined by the individual. Many sleep difficulties are secondary to, or a symptom of, physical or mental problems such as pain, thyroid problems, worry, excitement, acute psychosis, mania or depression, sleep apnea, stimulant drugs, drug dependence, or drug withdrawal. Other reasons for insomnia can be disruption in circadian rhythms or environmental changes. Not much is known about the neurochemical basis for insomnia (Wincor, 1990).

Treatment of insomnia depends on the type of insomnia. Assessing the sleep pattern is important in formulating an accurate diagnosis and selecting appropriate treatment. There is no ideal hypnotic drug or agent that induces sleep. Every marketed hypnotic has at least one of the following drawbacks:

- The individual is unable to maintain sleep for the expected duration.
- The individual is able to maintain sleep throughout the night but suffers a morning hangover effect.
- Problems associated with dependence and tolerance and with abrupt withdrawal of a hypnotic agent produces rebound insomnia.

Hypnotics should be avoided when possible in chronic insomnia because of their abuse potential. The only exception to this rule is a condition called *nocturnal myoclonus* wherein frequent muscle jerks produce "mini-arousals" during sleep (Wincor, 1990).

CLASSES OF HYPNOTIC AGENTS

Hypnotics produce a state of CNS depression resembling normal sleep. Utilizing smaller doses of hypnotic agents causes a state of drowsiness. When used in this manner, these agents are called *sedatives*. Progressive dose-related effects of hypnotics or sedatives are clear (Julien, 1996):

Most hypnotics are habit-forming; therefore short-term use (7 to 10 days) is recommended. One CNS depressant can be potentiated by other CNS depressants (alcohol or another hypnotic drug). Ingesting various CNS depressants together can be lethal!

BARBITURATES.   Barbiturates are a class of CNS depressant drugs that were frequently prescribed as sedatives. Barbiturates are not prescribed as often today because they

- have a narrow margin of safety
- have a moderately high abuse potential
- produce many drug interactions by induction of liver enzymes, and
- suppress both delta wave sleep and REM sleep

After use over 14 consecutive nights, barbiturates lose their sleep-inducing efficacy unless a higher dose is taken. Barbiturates exert their effect by interrupting impulses in the brain's reticular activating system (RAS), which is responsible for alertness and attention (Olin et al., 1998). The most common barbiturates are listed in Table 3-5.

BENZODIAZEPINES (BZDs).   BZDs are effective hypnotics. Compared to the barbiturates, BZDs are somewhat less likely to produce tolerance and physical dependence; however, tolerance, dependence, and addiction do develop, and the onset of dependence is often insidious. The client takes the medication to help with a light to moderate insomnia; however, if the drug is discontinued after several weeks of use, the client will probably have severe insomnia for

Table 3-5   Common Barbiturates

Trade Name	Generic Name
Amytal	amobarbital
Butisol	butabarbital
Luminal	phenobarbital
Mebaral	mephobarbital
Nembutal	pentobarbital
Seconal	secobarbital

Source: Olin et al., 1993.

several evenings. Thus, the drug both cures and causes sleep problems. Fortunately, most clients who abandon use of the drug do finally sleep.

These agents are usually not lethal unless taken in relatively large doses (great difference exists between toxic and therapeutic doses). Geriatric doses should be reduced from normal adult doses (Maxmen, 1991).

Mechanism of Action: BZDs act on the GABA (an important inhibitory CNS neurotransmitter) receptor complex by enhancing GABA's inhibitory (sedative) activity. BZDs usually decrease the period from retiring to sleep onset (latency) and decrease the number of awakenings. REM sleep is shortened by BZDs, and most BZDs suppress delta sleep (Wincor, 1990). Some common BZDs are listed in Table 3-6. Drowsiness, ataxia (defective muscular coordination), syncope (fainting), paradoxical excitement, rash, nausea, and altered libido are possible side effects of BZDs (Olin et al., 1998). BZDs can exacerbate a depressive illness in the elderly and may cause an increase in suicidal ideation (Wright, 1996).

Halcion, a triazolam, is used widely because it has the least effect on delta sleep and is least likely to produce morning hangover. However, it has been criticized for its potential to produce CNS problems, including: amnesia, anxiety, delusions, and hostility. Also, the unexpected effects it can produce

Table 3-6   Benzodiazepines (BZDs)

Trade Name	Generic Name
Dalmane	flurazepam
Doral	quazepam
Halcion	triazolam
ProSom	estazolam
Restoril	temazepam

(usually the drugs disinhibiting effects on impulse control) are often attributed to the individual instead of to the drug (Olin et al., 1998). Arguments about these effects and the client's legal responsibility for them have spawned a variety of lawsuits. Halcion is more helpful in assisting an individual with falling asleep than it is in sustaining a sleep state (Swonger & Matejski, 1991).

ANTIHISTAMINE HYPNOTICS.   Another group of hypnotic agents includes the *antihistamine hypnotics.* A useful side effect of some antihistamines is sedation. Because there is little physiological addiction potential, antihistamines are considered safe hypnotics. It should be remembered, however, that discontinuation of antihistamines after a long period of use will probably result in poor sleep for several nights until the body adjusts to the lack of drug in the system. The most popular antihistamine hypnotic is Benadryl. The adult dose as a sleep aid is 50 mg at bedtime. Patients subjectively report that the effect of Benadryl (50 mg) is equivalent to phenobarbital (60 mg). Increasing the dose of Benadryl does not increase its hypnotic effect, only its anticholinergic side effects.

Although hypnotics produce a state of CNS depression resembling sleep, it differs from normal sleep. Sleep induced by most sedative hypnotic drugs alters normal sleep stages and can affect dreams. Melatonin, a natural hormone secreted mostly at night in the brain, promotes sleep. It also promotes sleep at any time of the day. Older adults may have lower levels of melatonin due to lowered activity (usually calcification) of the pineal gland. Also, aspirin and ibuprofen inhibit normal production of melatonin. At a dose of 0.3 mg, melatonin has been effective in hastening onset of sleep. Melatonin is sold in health food stores and, unfortunately, is not regulated by the FDA. Often it is sold at doses ten times the dose that promotes normal sleep. When too much melatonin accumulates in the body, daytime drowsiness, dizziness, and nightmares may result (Grinspoon, 1996).

In addition to the classes of hypnotics we have discussed here, there are a number of miscellaneous hypnotics to consider. These are listed in Table 3-7. All these agents are DEA-controlled substances.

Table 3-7   Miscellaneous Hypnotic Agent

Trade Name	Generic Name
Ambien	zolpidem
Doriden	glutethimide
Noctec	chloral hydrate
Noludar	methyprylon
Paral	paraldehyde
Placidyl	ethchlorvynol

Source: Olin et al., 1993; Julien, 1998.

CHAPTER 3 REVIEW QUESTIONS

1. Describe the role of serotonin in anxiolytic medications.
2. What are the BZDs and what is their mode of action?
3. How might we best describe anxiety or panic in terms of receptors or neurochemicals?
4. Why should the elderly avoid using long-acting benzodiazepines?
5. Under what conditions is drug treatment for anxiety indicated and under what conditions is anxiety management therapy alone the treatment of choice?
6. What organic conditions are associated with panic and anxiety symptoms?
7. Describe short-term and long-term withdrawal symptoms from BZDs.
8. Under what conditions should anxious clients be referred for psychiatric evaluation for medication?
9. Describe the stages of sleep.
10. What are the most common sleep disorders and how are they treated?
11. What are the primary classes of hypnotic agents and how do they function to produce sleep?
12. Describe the most significant drug interactions that involve BZDs.

WEB RESOURCES ABOUT ANXIETY

In your Internet browser, either Netscape or Internet Explorer, there is a blank space available where you can type the following URL addresses. URL addresses are universal resource locations that start with the letters "http://" and show you a page of information on the Internet. Type any of the following URL addresses into that space and press return in order to go to that page. A variety of access buttons (highlighted words that you may point and click on) are available for further information.

Please note that because of the continuously changing sites, we cannot guarantee that pages will remain at their location address. If pages are incomplete, use the address without the last part of the extension (instead of using http://www.adaa.org/4_info/4__01.htm, use http://www.adaa.org/).

A. http://www.adaa.org/4_info/4__01.htm
What information does this URL address provide?
This page lists and describes the different types of anxiety disorders (Panic Disorders, Generalized Anxiety Disorders, Obsessive-Compulsive Disorders, Post-Traumatic Stress Disorders, and different phobias). It also addresses the variety of medications prescribed for anxiety disorders, how those medications are thought to work, and benefits and drawbacks of the medication (some examples of medications presented are Ativan, BuSpar, Nardil, Prozac, and Elavil). The page also includes information on different age groups with anxiety disorders and where one can go for support.

How can this page be used?

At the top of the page, a list of general topics is presented, the topic words are either presented in boxes or with underlines. To select a topic, click on it. For example, upon clicking the boxed topic "Helping a Family Member," a page appears with other topics like "Providing Support," and "Helping the Patient With Homework." Click on these topics to find out more information about them.

In the middle of the page, a variety of topics are presented. Click on these topics to find out specific information about the topic. Other topics will be available at those pages as well. For example, upon clicking on the topic "Generalized Anxiety Disorder," a page is displayed discussing the disorder. That page also includes other topics like "Finding Help" and "GAD Self-Help Test" that may be chosen by clicking the topic.

B. http://www.nimh.nih.gov/publicat/anxiety.htm

C. http://panicdisorder.miningco.com/msub21.htm

D. http://www.anxietynetwork.com/

WEB RESOURCES ABOUT SLEEP DISORDERS

In your Internet browser, either Netscape or Internet Explorer, there is a blank space available where you can type the following URL addresses. URL addresses are universal resource locations that start with the letters "http://" and show you a page of information on the Internet. Type any of the following URL addresses into that space and press return in order to go to that page. A variety of access buttons (highlighted words that you may point and click on) are available for further information.

Please note that because of the continuously changing sites, we cannot guarantee that pages will remain at their location address. If pages are incomplete, use the address without the last part of the extension (instead of using http://www.sleep-sdca.com/home.htm, use http://www.sleep-sdca.com/).

A. http://www-leland.stanford.edu/~dement/sleepinfo.html

What information does this URL address provide?

Various types of sleep disorders (such as insomnia and restless legs syndrome), sleep stage disorders (sleep intertia and sleep terrors), and sleep disorders associated with medical conditions are described. For each disorder, information about symptoms, treatment, prognosis, and other resources for support is made available.

How can this page be used?

In the middle of the page, types of disorders are listed in categories. Each disorder can be clicked on to locate further information. For example, under the Dyssomnias category, the topics "Advanced Sleep Phase Syndrome," "Delayed Sleep Phase Syndrome," and "Time Zone Change Syndrome — Jet Lag" are listed. Click on one of the topics for further information. Upon clicking on "Delayed Sleep Phase Syndrome," a page appears with further topics, such as

Symptoms   Treatment for DSPS
What Causes DSPS?   DSPS and Depression
Getting Help   Further Information/Links

Click on a topic for further information and other topics that may be available for clicking for further information. For example, upon clicking the "Symptoms" topic, a page appears with text about symptoms and the topics "How can DSPS be distinguished from other causes of insomnia, such as insomnia caused by stress or tension?" and "Why is it so hard for me to get up in the morning?"

B. http://www.sleepnet.com/disorder.htm#sleep1

C. http://www.users.cloud9.net/~thorpy/

D. http://www.sleep-sdca.com/home.htm

4

PSYCHOSIS AND THE ANTIPSYCHOTICS

The term *psychosis* was once used to describe any mental disorder but now represents a collection of mental disorders manifested by inabilities in perceiving and testing reality and in communicating effectively with others to the extent that the individual cannot meet everyday demands (Thomas, 1985). Psychotic behavior that follows from the mental disorder is often active but seemingly purposeless, inappropriate, abnormal, and sometimes threatening if challenged.

Chronic psychotic states can be subdivided into several major types that may not be mutually exclusive etiologically (e.g., causally). Schizophrenia, for example, is thought of today as an organic brain syndrome. These general subdivisions are:

- *organic brain syndromes*, which represent a loss or alteration in nerve cell functioning that can occur with dementia (including Alzheimer's, multiple sclerosis, autism, and AIDS) and drug intoxications
- *affective disorders*, including manic psychosis or depressive psychosis
- *schizophrenia*; and
- *schizoaffective disorders* (Andreasen, 1989)

Brief or transient psychoses, typical in delirium and substance abuse, are diagnostic in schizophreniform disorders and are common features in borderline and schizotypal personality disorders.

It is commonly held that various clinical manifestations of psychosis share some physiological pathways but not others. Whether schizoaffective disorder is classified as a subcategory of schizophrenia or as an affective disorder or as a separate, independent process is not clear. Even though there is no consensus, treatment experience and research data indicate that schizoaffective disorder should be included in the affective area (Silverstone, 1989). Support for this view derives from findings that clients with schizoaffective disorders, like bipolars, respond better to lithium treatment, whereas schizoaffective lithium nonresponders respond better to carbamazepine (CBZ: Tegretol, an anticonvulsant tricyclic) than to traditional schizophrenia drugs (variously referred to as **antipsychotics, neuroleptics,** or **major tranquilizers**) such as the phenothiazines or haloperidol (Brown & Herz, 1989; Okuma, 1989).

Sensitivity to antipsychotic medication has been proposed as a possible diagnostic criterion for schizophrenia, whereas nonsensitivity indicates schizoaffective disorder or some other disorder (Brown & Herz, 1989). The development of second generation drugs with a variety of antipsychotic effects has clouded this picture. [Additionally, some patients with affective or personality disorders, with clinical or subclinical psychotic features, respond favorably to a medication regimen that includes an antipsychotic.]

There have also been conflicting findings in attempts to establish the degree to which positive (hallucinatory) and negative (depressive) symptoms in this family of psychotic disorders are diagnostic. Even though depression is typically seen in schizophrenia and is frequently a side effect of traditional neuroleptic drug treatment, symptoms of schizophrenia do not remit when depression remits (Silverstone, 1989). Further, evidence from family genetic studies indicates a close etiological connection between schizophrenia and schizotypal and paranoid disorders (Andreasen, 1989; Baron et al., 1985).

Even though it is possible that neuroleptic-resistant clients do not have schizophrenia, many are simply given higher doses of neuroleptics to capitalize on the general tranquilizing effects of the drugs rather than being taken off the drugs completely during a reanalysis of the problem (Brown & Herz, 1989). Treatment implications for the psychotic and nonpsychotic disorders are presented in Table 4-1.

Traditional antipsychotics (phenothiazines) have been augmented in the past several years by what are usually referred to as "new generation" antipsychotics (clozapine, for example) that tend to work on several neurotransmitter systems, including a variety of dopamine, norepinephrine, and serotonin subreceptors. These new generation drugs will be explored in more detail subsequently, but it is important to understand that the physiological systems underlying psychotic disorders—schizophrenia, for example—are complex in expression and multisystemic in origin. Thus, psychoses can best be viewed as part of a syndrome in which many brain systems are involved, systems that have experienced varying degrees of incapacitation due to the extent, timing, and location of the particular organic insult or accident.

Table 4-1   Treatment Recommendations for Psychotic and Nonpsychotic Disorders

Disorder	Recommended Treatment
Psychotic Disorders	
Schizophrenia	Neuroleptics
Affective disorders (manic and depressive psychosis)	Lithium, Tegretol, antidepressants
Schizoaffective disorder	Lithium, Tegretol, antidepressants
Nonpsychotic Disorders	
Nonpsychotic schizophrenia spectrum disorder	Outpatient psychotherapy; usually not medicated
Schizotypal p.d.	
Schizoid p.d.	
Paranoid p.d.	
Nonpsychotic affective spectrum disorder	Outpatient psychotherapy
Borderline p.d. (variable: antidepressant, mood stabilizer, antipsychotic)	
Cyclothymic	
Dysthymic (antidepressant)	

Source: Andreasen, 1989.

Antipsychotic medications may be appropriate when any of these symptoms are present, including:

- schizophrenia
- mania
- psychosis
- acute agitation
- withdrawal hallucinosis (Olin et al., 1998)

Some antipsychotics cause useful side effects such as sedation, decreased anxiety, and mood elevation. However, if the patient's primary problem is insomnia, anxiety, or depression, antipsychotics should not be prescribed.

SCHIZOPHRENIA

Approximately 1% of the world's population suffer from schizophrenia (APA, 1994) and about half of the 175,000 patients in U.S. mental institutions have diagnoses of schizophrenia. Schizophrenia is a form of psychosis that apparently affects women and men and all ethnic groups equally. Early age of onset has been found to be an unfavorable prognostic feature in the illness. Mortality of victims is about twice the rate for individuals without schizophrenia, and the suicide rate within the first 10 years of diagnosis is approximately 10% (Allebeck, 1989; Julien, 1998). Between 15 and 50% of those with schizophrenia experience depression both prodromal (prior to onset) to acute exacerbations of the psychosis and after recovery (Heinrichs & Carpenter, 1985; Loebel et al., 1992; Marder et al., 1991; Siris et al., 1991). Thus, depression is a common cause of relapse into primary symptoms as well as a common result of relapse. Individuals with schizophrenia account for 500,000 hospitalizations each year (Bellack, 1989), most of which are in local community hospitals rather than in mental institutions. Of the 3 million homeless, approximately half are chronically mentally ill, and many have schizophrenia and cannot manage their own money or their own care.

Schizophrenia is a difficult illness to control with medications for many reasons. More than 20% of those with schizophrenia do not respond positively to antipsychotic medications, 30–50% refuse to take them for a variety of reasons, 20–30% relapse chronically even though they do comply with medical treatment, and approximately 30% experience significant, sometimes debilitating, side effects from the drugs (Bellack, 1989).

DIAGNOSIS OF SCHIZOPHRENIA

Schizophrenia is distinguished in DSM-IV (APA, 1994) by the following characteristics: (a) multiple psychiatric processes; (b) deterioration of functioning; (c) duration of over 6 months; (d) not due to affective disorder; and (e) delusions, hallucinations, and thought disturbances. DSM-IV divides schizophrenia into five general subtypes:

- *catatonic*, marked by decreased reactivity, posturing, or purposeless activity
- *disorganized*, marked by incoherent or incongruous affect without systematic delusions
- *paranoid*, marked by systematic delusions
- *residual*, marked by emotional blunting and loose associations without persistent delusions or hallucinations
- *undifferentiated*, not classifiable but hallucinations or delusions are clearly present

Another way to characterize the disease of schizophrenia is by globally categorizing symptoms into two groups:

- Positive symptoms include *thought disorder*, evidenced by delusions, beliefs that are contrary to facts, and hallucinations, wherein an individual perceives something, usually auditory, that is not present, *disorganized speech or behavior*, and *catatonic behavior*, such as excessive or absent motor activity.
- Negative symptoms include flattened emotional response, poverty of speech, lack of initiative, and persistent inability to experience pleasure. This constellation of symptoms is also seen in individuals who have endured damage to the frontal lobe of the brain (Price & Lynn, 1986) and is resistant to traditional neuroleptic treatment. These symptoms are less resistant to the new generation drugs, and the new drugs have begun to revolutionize the treat-

ment of schizophrenia and other psychotic disorders much as the phenothiazines revolutionized the treatment of schizophrenia in the 1950s.

This dichotomy in symptom categorization into positive and negative suggests that different biochemical and neurological disorders may produce schizophrenia. Most individuals with schizophrenia have a combination of positive and negative symptoms. Positive symptoms are usually alleviated by drug treatment, which decreases action at dopamine-2 receptors. Effects of this drug treatment tend to confirm that the positive symptoms are due to overactivity at dopamine-2 receptors (and probably other dopamine receptors and autoreceptors as well: Price & Lynn, 1986), while the negative, generally depressive symptoms appear to result from abnormalities at 5-HT2 receptors. Finally, other neurotransmitter systems may be affected in psychotic disorders, especially disorders with a progressive and deteriorating course.

DOPAMINE HYPOTHESIS

The **dopamine hypothesis** of the cause of schizophrenia or psychoses states that the positive signs of schizophrenia are due to overactivity of dopamine in the brain's mesolimbic system (Leccese, 1991). General evidence in support of the dopamine hypothesis stems from factors found to be important in the treatment of Parkinson's disease. In Parkinson's, dopaminergic neurons in the brain's substantia nigra are affected. Exogenous dopamine, given in the form of L-dopa, is administered to increase CNS dopamine activity. Although the exogenous dopamine may improve Parkinson symptoms, an unwanted side effect that sometimes develops with the use of L-dopa is schizophrenia-like behavior (Olin et al., 1998). Other drugs that increase the availability of CNS dopamine are also known to produce positive symptoms of schizophrenia— for example, the psychotomimetic agents cocaine and amphetamine. Finally, lysergic acid diethylamide (LSD) and phencyclidine (PCP) are both known psychotomimetics, and their use is often associated with exacerbations of schizophrenia.

In conclusion, today schizophrenia is thought to be a developmental brain disorder that is strongly influenced by genetic factors. An inherited lack of fetal resistance to viral and other teratogenic factors during the first trimester of pregnancy may account for a variety of brain system injuries that are responsible for the complex syndrome of phenotypic features that make up the schizophrenic and other psychotic syndromes.

TREATMENT OF SCHIZOPHRENIA

Like many of the major psychiatric illnesses, a **stress-diathesis model** (stress and underlying biological factors) has been proposed for the onset of and relapse into psychosis. Even though it is clear that schizophrenia is caused by organic factors that necessitate lifelong adaptation, the chronicity or life history of the disease for each person is greatly affected by stressors from the external environment. Lack of a stable home, family support, meaningful work, and worthwhile community involvement are typical external stressors. At the same time, psychological resilience is influenced as well by community-controlled factors that negate some stressors, such as continuing education, counseling, and crisis intervention.

The instability of mood, disorganization in thought processes, and eccentricities of behavior among those with schizophrenia often cause them to feel socially inadequate, particularly in their family environment if family members are hypervigilant and intrusive. This social distress adds to normal life stress, and the cumulative burden leads to negative psychological consequences, including low self-esteem and self-efficacy, social withdrawal, loneliness, boredom, and affective difficulties such as depression and anxiety.

Stress, depression, and anxiety are sufficient to cause an exacerbation or relapse of psychotic symptoms. Continued stress leads to chronicity. Chronicity exacerbates both positive and negative symptoms of the illness. And failure to manage symptoms effectively continues the cycle of rejection, relapse, and acting out.

RELAPSE.   Contemporary therapy for those with schizophrenia emphasizes the role for neuroleptic drugs, the family, the community, and ongoing individual therapy in modifying the stress conditions that lead to relapse (Kane, 1989). Conditions that should alert therapists to a probability of relapse are

- increases in either positive or negative symptoms (20 to 50% experience depression prior to exacerbations)
- major stressors (including changes in living or job situation, familial intrusions or losses, changes in medications—compliance failure or reduction of dose, change in physician or therapist)
- use of alcohol or illicit drugs
- physiological problems
- problems with the legal system (20 to 30% have been incarcerated)
- changes in global assessment of functioning (GAF) as defined in the DSM-IV, or
- denial that the underlying illness is still present. (Kane, 1989; Marder et al., 1991)

Heinrichs and Carpenter (1985) provide the following list of late-prodromal symptoms and their relative frequency during relapse (decompensation) of 47 patients with schizophrenia: hallucinations (53%), suspiciousness (43%), change in sleep pattern (43%), anxiety (38%), cognitive inefficiency (26%), anger/hostility (23%), somatic symptoms or delusions (21%), thought disorder (17%), disruptive inappropriate behavior (17%), and depression (17%). Finally, Marder et al. (1991) found that even relatively small changes in emotional-behavioral signs and symptoms in maintenance treatment for schizophrenia might be clinically meaningful.

GENDER DIFFERENCES.   Researchers have found that when the confounding factors of age and marital status are controlled for, women with schizophrenia have a better prognosis in hospital treatment, experience shorter hospitalization, and survive longer in the community after their first hospital admission than do men (Angermeyer, Kuhn, & Goldstein, 1990). Moreover, Angermeyer et al. (1990) found evidence that men are hospitalized earlier than women and that the onset of the disorder is earlier among men. Thus, for reasons that are unclear but that may relate to the prophylactic effects of higher estrogen levels, the course of schizophrenia is milder and social adaptation is better among women. Further, more women were involved in parenting their children, were more likely to be heterosexually active, and were more likely to be living with a partner of the opposite sex (Test, Burke, & Wallisch, 1990). However, this significant positive difference should not mislead therapists to believe that the course for particular female clients will be better. Unfortunately, as women age, their relapse histories mirror those of their male counterparts (Angermeyer et al., 1990).

CHILDREN.   Few studies of the efficacy of antipsychotics in the treatment of psychoses among children have been undertaken (Gadow, 1992). One double-blind placebo-controlled study reported in Spencer et al. (1992) showed that haloperidol (Haldol) and loxapine (Loxitane) were superior to a placebo in controlling psychotic symptoms in children with schizophrenia. Spencer et al. (1992) found that haloperidol was effective enough and had limited enough side effects among a small group of hospitalized children with schizophrenia that they were able to continue on the medication after discharge. Side effects, including akathesia, neuroleptic malignant syndrome, and tardive dyskinesia are more likely among children with developmental disabilities than among other psychotic children. Even with proper dosage, neuroleptics are known to reach toxic levels quickly in children and to induce a variety of affective and behavioral problems (Gadow, 1992). Therefore, their use should always be closely monitored by a professional who specializes in child psychiatry. The second generation antipsychotic medications offer more hope than the traditional ones for children with psychotic disorders because their side-effect profiles are less negative and their effects on physical development and motor coordination are less profound.

DEPRESSION IN SCHIZOPHRENIA.   Because anxiety and depression are of particular importance to therapists who work with clients with schizophrenia, the following guidelines suggested by Johnson (1989) are presented to increase a practical understanding and approach to the relationship between psychosis and depression.

1. Overall, one-third of depressions among psychotics who are not having psychotic symptoms remit within 2 months without any change in treatment. The proportion is higher during the postpsychotic period.
2. The emergence of new depressive symptoms during remission of psychosis, particularly after an interval of 1 year, indicates incipient relapse.
3. Approximately 10–15% of depressed clients on maintenance neuroleptics suffer from akinetic syndrome (muscular movement disorder), which responds to anticholinergic medication.
4. Pharmacogenic (drug-induced) depression must be considered. Dose reduction or change in drug regimen must be considered.
5. Because tricyclic antidepressants often increase deterioration in those with schizophrenia, they should be used cautiously and closely monitored. Although research is lacking in this area, SSRIs and atypical antidepressants may prove more useful.
6. Clinical research into the uses of lithium present conflicting results; however, a therapeutic trial with patients with recurrent depressions may be useful. This is especially true if features of mania are present.
7. Minor tranquilizers given for agitation accompanying depression may cause the underlying psychosis to arise.

PSYCHOTHERAPY. In addition to playing active roles in the emergency mental health networks in their communities, therapists in community mental health centers, medical settings, and private practice routinely play an important part in helping clients with schizophrenia adapt to life through consultation, psychotherapy, education, and referral. An understanding of the disease process itself as well as the neuroleptic medications for schizophrenia (and those used in conjunction to treat the affective components—anxiolytics and antidepressants) is crucial in this effort. As Coursey (1989) has said, "[Individuals with schizophrenia] desperately need to understand what causes their disability and what does not, what intensifies their symptoms, and what their prognosis might be" (p. 350). Further, Coursey identified three important domains amenable to psychotherapy. First, psychological issues raised by the disorders that disturb core psychological functions (identity and efficacy, for example). Second, illness-related problems clients can learn to better self-manage (diabetes, for example). And third, human problems that are not specific to schizophrenia but that require special attention because of the client's condition.

Although counselors, especially those who work with the chronically mentally ill, routinely take a case management approach, Coursey (1989) reasonably argues that therapists should use counseling skills rather than rely primarily on social work case management skills. Much like counseling the dying involves helping clients come to terms with death, the primary focus of psychotherapy among those with schizophrenia is not, important as it may be, to prevent relapse. Rather, counseling helps clients come to terms with the life experience and meaning of the disease. Although Coursey's view is well taken, it is important to note that psychotherapy cannot take place while clients are decompensating. Therefore, therapists must take a multifaceted approach in working with clients with schizophrenia.

It is also important that therapists realize, contrary to the way many comparative research projects are framed, that medications and psychotherapy are complementary. Complementarity is important to emphasize in working with individuals for whom prophylactic drug use is so pervasive and where side effects are often profound and permanent. Fortunately for clients who are refractory to drug treatment, cognitive-behavioral and psychosocial strategies are often successful in supporting remission (Brenner et al., 1990).

SCHIZOPHRENIA CASE STUDY

Nila, a 57-year-old, Asian-American woman arrived at the local community mental health center for an intake assessment following her first psychiatric hospitalization. She came to the attention of the mental health authorities 3 months prior, when her 14-year-old son was picked up for a curfew violation. Her son had reluctantly disclosed to a social worker from children's services that his mother, while always different, had been acting in an increasingly bizarre manner. He reported that during the prior week, she had begun taking off her clothes in the living room and then standing on the stove naked making declarations about the FBI bugging the apartment and telling her son it was not safe for him to go to school. The state office of children's services contacted his married sister and placed him temporarily in her custody. A social worker and the police found Nila in her apartment, unkempt, paranoid, and argumentative. She declined to answer any questions and talked in a rambling manner about the forces of evil and being spied on by the FBI. She reported carrying a gun in her purse for safety from imaginary persecutors. She stated that if she could afford to purchase Kryptonite everything would be all right.

The social worker persuaded Nila to undergo an emergency psychiatric evaluation, which resulted in her commitment to the state hospital, where she was diagnosed with schizophrenia, paranoid type. More typically diagnosed in early adulthood, individuals with schizophrenia have usually come to the attention of the social services system much earlier than Nila. Nila received an initial injection of Haldol, an antipsychotic, followed by daily oral Haldol. She briefly became more cooperative and less agitated.

After 2 weeks of taking the medication, Nila began pretending to take the Haldol by holding it in her cheek. She resumed her initial suspicious, haughty, and demanding manner and did not make any therapeutic gains over several weeks. Closer observation by the nursing staff revealed Nila's pretense and untaken pills in her locker. The psychiatrist changed her medication to a long-acting form of injectable Haldol, Haldol decanoate, often referred to as Haldol D.

During her 3 months at the state hospital, Nila attended daily group and weekly individual therapy and participated in recreational and work therapy activities as well. Therapists worked to improve her social functioning and help her regain a routine and carry out necessary daily activities. Nila remained paranoid and socially aloof. She reported enjoying talking with peers while they carried out simple tasks in the cafeteria. Developing more than superficial insight into her schizophrenia proved to be an unrealistic goal in Nila's case because of the distancing her paranoid personality engendered.

In the course of discharge planning from the hospital, it became apparent that Nila's family was frightened of her and unwilling for her to live at home. Family therapy was deferred until postdischarge because her family lived 2 hours from the hospital. Nila was released to live in a supervised apartment complex for persons with serious and persistent mental illnesses (SPMI). She came to the community mental health center with the recommendation from the hospital staff that she receive some family assessment and psychoeduca-tion sessions, psychiatric follow-up, case management, and a weekly group therapy session for persons with schizophrenia.

When she and her outpatient therapist met, Nila was well groomed, soft-spoken, and pleasant. She spoke in a flat tone of voice and her affect was blunted. She was, however, alert and oriented, even though her speech was often vague and tangential. She seemed unclear about the events surrounding her hospitalization and avoided important topics, such as losing custody of her son. Because she lacked insight into her illness and was considered likely to be noncompliant with medication, biweekly Haldol injections were continued. Nila told her outpatient therapist her main goal was to find a regular job.

An important goal of family therapy is to provide psychoeducation about accepting and living with or near a family member with schizophrenia. Per-sons with schizophrenia cope much better in interpersonal environments that are calm, supportive, respectful, consistent, and well structured. Further, clients do better when they are able to participate in productive work, whether paid or voluntary. Even though clients need to focus on realistic expectations and are helped to identify short-term, concrete goals and behaviors, it is also important not to squelch long-term goals and dreams. Irrational expectations, however, must give way to such mundane considerations as getting up at a regular time, bathing daily, and finding a low-stress job before more long-term goals can be realistically assessed. Keeping in mind Nila's desire to find full-time employment, for example, her therapist might ask her what she needs to do today, this week, and this month to work toward her goal.

Because Nila retained a high level of residual paranoia, her outpatient therapist decided to have Nila present at family education sessions. Nila's son was still fearful of her and was not ready to talk about his experiences living with his mother when she was psychotic. He did not attend the first family education session with Nila and her daughter. Early in the session, Nila agreed to sell her gun and agreed to have a case manager observe her take her medication daily. She also agreed that the case manager would bring her to the community mental health center for any appointments. The therapist worked with Nila's daughter to plan a series of brief low-stress outings to provide a forum for Nila to interact with her son in settings where he was likely to feel safe and in control. Nila's son would be invited to attend subsequent sessions but was given support not to exceed his comfort level.

Her outpatient therapist provided Nila and her daughter with educational materials outlining measures that clients and families have found helpful in preventing relapse and normalizing family relations to the greatest extent possible. Highlights include: (a) creating a low-stress environment; (b) having a structured format for resolving disagreements; (c) learning to take time out from discussions if emotions are rising and creative problem solving is declining; (d) not arguing with clients about unrealistic expectations but helping them identify concrete, realistic short-term goals; (e) planning both group and individual activities; (f) treating one another with respect; and (g) seeking help when stuck. Having handouts to review and to share with other family members offers a simple way to help increase the impact of education sessions.

Nila's case brings up several other important points about the complementary role of therapy for clients taking medication for schizophrenia. First, medication could not help Nila deal with her grief about losing custody of her son. It might, however, stabilize her to the point that she could explore her grief and loss if she chose to do so. Second, even though Nila accomplished much because of her medication regimen, good communication between staff and careful discharge planning proved crucial. Explaining to Nila what was happening and what to expect during the first weeks of discharge and involving her daughter early in the discharge-planning process were important to limiting Nila's anxiety and giving her a sense of predictability. Outpatient therapy can assist clients like Nila (a) manage symptoms and a treatment regime within the least restrictive environment needed for basic safety, (b) improve relationships with self and with others, (c) cope with feelings about having a mental illness and needing medication, and (d) work on issues of identity and self-esteem (see Coursey, 1989).

ANTIPSYCHOTIC DRUG ACTION

Terms used to describe the general category of antipsychotic drugs include *major tranquilizers, neuroleptics, antischizophrenics, psychostatics,* and **psychotropics**. Today, the term *neuroleptic* is principally used to indicate the phenothiazine drugs and Haldol that are used to treat the positive symptoms of schizophrenia, while *newer* or *second generation* is used to describe more current, multiaction medications. All antipsychotics, new and traditional, block or reregulate dopamine (D2) receptors in the brain, thereby preventing dopamine from exerting its maximum effect.

The first drugs to successfully treat psychoses were introduced in the early 1950s after it was discovered that phenothiazine drugs used experimentally to decrease anxiety prior to surgery produced a profoundly calm and disinterested condition. This condition was later referred to as a **neuroleptic state**. It was soon noted that these drugs—first, promethazine and chlorpromazine (Thorazine) and later Haldol and Mellaril—also produced negative neurological effects represented by a constellation of unwanted motor movements when administered to psychiatric patients. The term *neuroleptic* derives from the neurological syndrome of movement problems characterizing these original antipsychotics. As we have indicated, this early group of antipsychotics is sometimes referred to as "typical" or traditional antipsychotics. Now, newer agents used in treatment of psychoses are atypical or second-generation antipsychotics. Clozaril (clozapine) and Zyprexa (olanzapine) are examples. At normal doses, atypical antipsychotics do not produce significant motor problems. Their multifaceted therapeutic action may be explained by their effects on both the serotonin and dopamine systems (Lacro & Kodsi, 1996). Recent developments in prescribing antipsychotic medications more often utilize smaller doses of the older (typical) antipsychotics and newer atypical antipsychotics together for treatment-resistant patients (Lacro & Kodsi, 1996).

THERAPEUTIC EFFECTS

Antipsychotics, principally the phenothiazines, induce in schizophrenia what we have referred to as the neuroleptic state, which is characterized by

> *psychomotor slowing* (decreased agitation, aggression, and impulsiveness),
> *decreased hallucinations and delusions,*
> *emotional quieting*, and
> *affective indifference* (not as concerned with external environment and not as easily aroused)

Symptoms likely to improve are combativeness, tension, hyperactivity, hostility, and hallucinations. Delusions may or may not improve. Symptoms that are not likely to improve are insight, judgment, and memory. Antipsychotics will help normalize sleep problems associated with many of the psychoses (Baldessarini, 1993). However, when administered to normal or asymptomatic individuals, antipsychotics may cause dysphoric or unpleasant effects (Julien, 1998). Consistent with the differences in chemical structure within the broad grouping of antipsychotics, these agents also differ in potencies and side effects (Ponterotto, 1985). The best prognosis for a patient taking antipsychotics is given to an individual with an acute psychotic episode who has a history of a healthy personality (Baldessarini, 1993) and a relatively short history of prodromal psychotic symptoms (Loebel et al., 1992).

SIDE EFFECTS

It usually takes 2 or more weeks for the drug's desired effect to occur, but side effects are often noticed sooner. Individuals taking antipsychotics must be warned about the delay of therapeutic effects. Adverse effects of antipsychotics are listed in Box 4-1. Extrapyramidal side effects are explained in detail in the list that follows.

Drug-induced movement disorders are associated with older classes of antipsychotic medications, especially the phenothiazines, including Thorazine, and the thioxanthenes. Treatment of these unwanted side effects consists primarily of antiparkinson medications, including, for example, benztropine and trihexyphenidyl. Anticholinergic treatment, however, that ordinarily produces dry mouth, dry skin, urinary retention, and blurred vision, can also cause negative effects on behavior and mental state. Unfortunately, even though anticholinergics can help reduce some movement disorder symptoms, they have been implicated as risk factors in tardive dyskinesia and in the exacerbation of psychotic symptoms.

Parkinsonian symptoms are marked by rigidity and limited movement and are evidenced by **akinesia** (complete or partial loss of muscle movement), muscle rigidity, shuffling gait, drooling, masklike facial expression, and tremor of extremities, especially the hands.

Box 4-1   Adverse Effects of Traditional Antipsychotics

Extrapyramidal Effects
Parkinsonian symptoms
Dystonic reactions
Akathisia
Dyskinesia
Tardive dyskinesia

Anticholinergic Effects
Dry mouth
Constipation
Blurred near vision
Urinary retention
Delayed ejaculation

CNS Effects
Sedation
Toxic psychosis
Seizures

Cardiovascular Effects
Orthostatic hypotension
EKG changes

Endocrine Effects
Amenorrhea (halt in menstruation)
Galactorrhea (breast milk production)
Gynecomastia (breast development)
Weight gain

Pigmentation Effects
Corneal, lenticular
Retinopathy
Skin

Allergic Effects
Hematologic
Skin
Hepatic

Source: Olin et al., 1993.

Dystonic reactions are involuntary and inappropriate postures and are evidenced by oculogyric crisis (fixed upward stare), torticollis (unilateral spasm of neck muscles), opisthotonos (arched back), and trismus, laryngospasm (spasm of muscles in jaw or throat).

Akathisia is manifested as a compulsion to move (fidgetiness) and an individual in constant motion, exhibiting motor restlessness, an inability to sit or stand still, or rocking and shifting weight while standing.

Dyskinesia is inappropriate motor movement appearing early in treatment and is evidenced by rhythmic clonic musculature contractions such as spasms, tics, and involuntary muscle movements.

Tardive dyskinesia is manifested by a rhythmical, involuntary movement of tongue, lips, or jaw, choreiform movements of extremities (jerky, purposeless movements), or athetoid movements of extremities, which are writhing, wormlike movements (Thomas, 1985; Olin et al., 1998).

Tardive dyskinesia (TD) is a syndrome of extrapyramidal side effects not uncommon with the use of traditional antipsychotics. Symptoms of tardive dyskinesia are similar to those of dyskinesia except that they occur later in drug therapy. This late-appearing side effect is characterized by abnormal, involuntary movements of the mouth, face, limbs, and trunk. Ten percent of the patients treated with antipsychotics develop TD (Julien, 1998). Among the chronically mentally ill, 26% of inpatients experience TD. Onset of TD is thought to be related to the patient's age and the drug's dose. Also, women are more likely than men to develop TD. Because TD is a potentially irreversible condition and its prevalence is increasing, antipsychotics should only be administered in appropriate situations. Additionally, because TD is dose related, discovering a minimum effective dose is important (Jeste & Wyatt, 1982).

A very serious complication that can occur when using antipsychotic agents, especially the phenothiazines and haloperidol, is **neuroleptic malignant syndrome** (NMS). NMS is like a severe form of Parkinson's, where the patient is catatonic (unable to move). Unstable blood pressure and heart rate, hyperthermia, mutism, and stupor are also part of this syndrome. Because NMS is sometimes fatal, intensive care is recommended. NMS is more likely to occur if the patient is also medically sick or has been taking many different antipsychotics, a situation referred to as **polypharmacy** (Caroff & Mann, 1988). After onset of NMS, the antipsychotic drug regimen is immediately discontinued. Following a single occurrence and recovery from NMS, there is an 80% chance of NMS reoccurring with the reintroduction of antipsychotics (Olin et al., 1998).

DRUG INTERACTIONS AND TOXICITY

The fact that antipsychotics generally have a large therapeutic window, meaning the toxic dose is much greater than the therapeutic dose, makes them relatively safe drugs. Undesirable side effects of antipsychotic agents render these drugs nonreinforcing. Therefore, this class of drugs is not likely to be abused (Baldessarini, 1993).

Because many of the traditional antipsychotics are highly protein-bound and remain in the bloodstream for a long time, the chance of interaction with other drugs is considerable (Olin et al., 1998). When selecting an antipsychotic agent, these factors should be considered:

- side-effect profile
- history of previous response
- dosage forms
- need for sedation
- other medication patient takes
- presence of physical disease
- patient compliance
- patient's sex and body weight
- stage and severity of the illness

Psychiatrists generally go through a "trial-and-error" ritual in prescribing antipsychotic agents.

CLASSIFICATION OF ANTIPSYCHOTIC DRUGS

PHENOTHIAZINES

All drugs in this category share the same basic chemical structure. Of all the antipsychotics, the **phenothiazines** are the oldest and the most prescribed (Ponterotto, 1985). Certain phenothiazines are used as antiemetics (antivomiting) and have other labeled uses; many have unlabeled uses. Some agents are marketed under more than one trade name. Phenothiazines act at dopamine-1 and dopamine-2 receptors. The onset of therapeutic action is delayed, usually requiring 4 to 6 weeks for maximum neuroleptic effect (Olin et al., 1998). Some of the more popular phenothiazines include

Trade Name	Generic Name
Compazine	prochlorperazine
Mellaril	thioridazine
Permitil	fluphenazine
Prolixin	fluphenazine
Serentil	mezoridazine
Sparine	promazine
Stelazine	trifluoperazine
Thorazine	chlorpromazine
Tindal	acetophenazine maleate
Trilafon	perphenazine
Vesprin	triflupromazine (Olin et al., 1998)

THIOXANTHENES AND BUTYROPHENONES

Haldoperidol (Haldol) and droperidol, both butyrophenones and developed in Europe in the 1960s, are structurally and functionally similar to the phenothiazines and have many of the same negative side effects. Haldol is the most potent of all the neuroleptics. It acts predominantly at dopamine-2 receptors. Haldol's adverse effects are primarily extrapyramidal side effects (EPS). Of all the antipsychotics, its EPS are the greatest. Other labeled uses of Haldol include: (1) Tourette's disorder; (2) severe behavioral problems in children such as combative explosive behavior that is unexplained by provocation; and (3) short-term use for hyperactive children. Anecdotal and unconfirmed evidence has surfaced that Asians may be more sensitive to this drug or are at higher risk for serious side effects or toxic reactions.

The chemical structure and effects of thioxanthenes, very potent and effective agents, are similar to those of phenothiazines (Baldessarini, 1993). The most common thioxanthenes include Navane (thiothixene) and Taractan (chlorprothixene). Loxitane (loxapine) is similar to the phenothiazines (Olin et al., 1998). Moban (molindone), also very similar, produces less sedation than the other drugs in this category.

SECOND GENERATION AND NEWER ANTIPSYCHOTIC DRUGS

The second generation antipsychotics are of increasing importance because they are effective without the same level of risk for neuroleptic syndrome and because they are effective in combatting the negative symptoms associated with schizophrenia and other psychoses. They include the following drugs:

Trade Name	Generic Name
Clozaril	clozapine
Risperdal	risperidone
Serlect	sertindole
Seroquel	quietapine
Zyprexa	olanzapine

The newer antipsychotic agents have many advantages over the older ones. They are less likely to cause extrapyramidal symptoms (movement disorder), they improve the negative symptoms of schizophrenia (impoverished speech, social withdrawal, blunt affect, and decreased motivation), and they are associated with a lower incidence of anticholinergic effects (dry mouth, blurred vision, and constipation). Pharmaceutical companies continually work to develop more effective and safer antipsychotic agents not only because the market is large and the demand stable but because the new generations of antipsychosis drugs are finding uses in other domains, including bipolar disorder and other organic brain syndromes, including Alzheimer's disease.

CLOZARIL (CLOZAPINE).   Clozaril is chemically similar to loxapine but is considered to be an atypical antipsychotic agent. Clozaril principally acts on dopamine-1 and serotonin receptors. Side effects are mainly anticholinergic. Also, there is a risk of seizures, and weight gain is common. Because of a serious, potentially fatal adverse effect called *agranulocytosis*, a restriction in the inability of bone marrow to produce white blood cells, Clozaril is not the drug of first choice in treating schizophrenia and must be prescribed with caution. Patients taking Clozaril must have weekly blood tests, especially early in their treatment regimen, to detect the possible onset of agranulocytosis (Brenner et al., 1990; Olin et al., 1998). By itself, Clozaril is an extremely expensive drug, costing over $4,000 annually. With the cost of the physician monitoring added, the price can quickly soar out of the reach of many needy patients (Wallis & Willwerth, 1992).

SEROQUEL (QUETIAPINE FUMARATE).   This is a new generation antipsychotic introduced in the fall of 1997. Although it affects multiple dopamine and serotonin neurotransmitter systems in the brain, the exact mechanism of action is unknown. Common adverse reactions with Seroquel include dizziness and drowsiness, and side effects associated with older antipsychotics (e.g., movement disorders) have been noted. Seroquel, however, offers the advantage of less weight gain compared to older antipsychotics (Olin et al., 1998; Saklad, 1997). Studies also suggest that Seroquel may be particularly effective in reducing aggression. In addition to affecting those with schizophrenia, it has been found to reduce psychotic symptoms among the elderly and among clients with depression and bipolar disorders ("Quetiapine," *Psychopharmacology Update*, May, 1998).

RISPERDAL (RISPERIDONE).   A unique antipsychotic, Risperdal was approved by the FDA in late 1993. Its mechanism of action is not fully understood but, like most of the second generation antipsychotics, it is thought to impact both serotonin and dopamine systems in the brain. Side effects, which do not include the high risk of movement disorder, include sleeplessness, nervousness, agitation, headaches, constipation, and nausea. Because Risperdal can impair judgement, thinking and motor skills, caution must be exercised when operating machinery. When taking Risperdal, use of sunscreen or protective clothing is advised. Like many other drugs, Risperdal can increase one's sensitivity to sunlight, causing one to burn easily. Alcohol should also be avoided.

ZYPREXA (OLANZAPINE).   Zyprexa is one of the newer antipsychotic agents. It's exact mechanism of action is not completely understood but its therapeutic effects are related to it's affinity for binding with serotonin and dopamine receptors. Possible side effects include headaches, dizziness, decrease in blood pressure, sleeplessness, nervousness, restlessness, agitation, anxiety, and hostility. The occurrence of other unwanted effects are dose related, meaning that as the dose of Zyprexa increases, the incidence of side effects increases.

Zyprexa's dose-related adverse effects include tremor, rigid muscles, drowsiness, and weakness. However, some unwanted actions such as drowsiness and constipation may decrease with time, while others such as weight gain may worsen. As with Risperdal, Zyprexa can impair judgement and motor skills, so caution is strongly advised when using machinery. Alcohol should be avoided while taking Zyprexa or any other antipsychotic medication (Olin et al., 1998; Schilli, 1996). Zyprexa's complex effects demonstrate the need for therapists to increase their knowledge about psychotropic medications. The case of G.R., a 31-year-old male, illustrates this problem.

G.R. was started on Zyprexa and his family noted significant improvement in his functioning within a week. However, on day 16 of drug treatment, he discontinued intake without consulting his family or physician. G.R. stated to his therapist that he was tired of feeling sleepy during the day. Unfortunately, G.R.'s therapist did not bring his family into therapy to discuss his actions. Within a week of stopping Zyprexa, G.R. started reexperiencing his thought disorder and his general condition worsened. Because of his confusion and growing paranoia, G.R. was unwilling to seek medical advice and his family had him hospitalized. This example illustrates several related concerns, including:

1. The need for very close client monitoring and communication between therapist and physician, especially during the first months of medication when side effects are most discouraging and most likely to lead to noncompliance
2. The need for consistent education of the client and family around compliance and relapse issues and around side-effect profiles of particular drugs
3. Ongoing contact among therapist, physician, and patient's family; it is usually the family who first notice medication noncompliance and negative effects on the patient's quality of life
4. The development of a relapse prevention plan as a normal part of patient-physician-therapist interaction

When clients complain about unwanted effects of their medication, therapists should faciliate contact with their doctor to obtain necessary information but also provide emotional support. If they have contacted their doctor or pharmacist and have knowledge that the side effects are not dangerous, clients need their therapist's encouragement in tolerating their medications' unwanted effects, establishing better interpersonal adaptation, and gaining employment when feasible.

ANTI-PARKINSON AGENTS

Anti-Parkinson agents are often prescribed to counteract drug-induced extrapyramidal, Parkinson's-like effects of the phenothiazines and Haldol. Among the drugs in this category are:

Trade Name	Generic Name
Akineton	biperiden
Artane	trihexyphenidyl
Benadryl	diphenhydramine
Cogentin	benztropine
Kemadrin	procyclidine
Parsidol	ethopropazine
Symmetrel	amantadine (Olin et al., 1998)

DRUGS THAT CAN PRODUCE PSYCHOTIC SYMPTOMS

Psychotic behavior is generally thought to result from a **functional disorder**, as in schizophrenia or depression. **Functional psychoses** are abnormal behaviors that cannot be attributed to any single known cause, whereas **organic psychoses** can result from a recognized insult to the brain, such as high fever or drug use (Price & Lynn, 1986). Almost every known drug has the potential to produce side effects that are manifested as psychotic behavior. Unfortunately, this abnormal behavior is often misdiagnosed as a functional disorder. The difficulty in making an accurate diagnosis coincides with the increase in both illicit drug use and self-medication. Not only is the increase in illicit drug consumption a problem but the underreporting in usage of both over-the-counter medication and prescription drugs adds to the confusion (Taylor, 1990). Additionally, separating drug side effects from the symptoms of the illness for which the therapeutic agent is administered can be challenging. In this section we discuss therapeutic agents, which are common or are known for the severity of their side effects.

PSYCHOTOXIC DRUGS

Psychotoxic drugs alter the functioning of the central nervous system (CNS). Baldessarini (1985) divides psychotoxic drugs into three subcategories:

1. Therapeutic agents that have legitimate uses but also possess a significant potential for abuse. Drugs in this category include sedatives, stimulants, and opioid analgesics.
2. Drugs that have no established medical use but are popular in today's society. Examples in this group are caffeine, alcohol, tobacco, marijuana, and hallucinogens.
3. Drugs that are valued for their medicinal benefits but that produce psychiatric side effects. Cardiac glycosides, antihypertensives, sedatives, stimulants, and steroids are members of this category.

We will not discuss drugs such as caffeine, tobacco, or others in the second grouping that lack any medically recognized benefits. Therapeutic agents with the potential for psychiatric adverse effects will be the focus. However,

Baldessarini's (1985) third category will be expanded. Drugs included in this grouping *directly affect* the CNS to produce psychotic behavior. We would be remiss if we omitted drugs that *indirectly alter* normal CNS functioning, such as agents that modify blood sugar levels or drugs that reduce cerebral blood flow. Therefore, we have also included drugs that indirectly alter CNS functioning.

SIDE EFFECTS.   Drug therapy should not be initiated unless the anticipated benefits outweigh the drug's potential hazards. Although the drug industry and the health community have made strides in increasing the reporting of adverse reactions, it is impossible to determine the exact probability or frequency of occurrence of a side effect. A higher incidence of adverse reactions has been reported among special populations, including females, geriatrics, children, and patients with kidney problems (Tatro, Ow-Wing, & Huie, 1986).

Side effects generally result from the agent's nonselective receptor-binding capacity. A drug circulating in the body will bind with any receptor that the drug's chemical structure will allow. Most therapeutic agents exert effects at other receptors in addition to the targeted receptor site. The majority of adverse effects are dose related, meaning as the dose increases, the number of side effects will also increase. Conversely, a decrease in dose usually decreases the magnitude of unwanted effects.

An **idiosyncratic reaction** is a type of side effect that occurs in only a very small percentage of the population. The exact mechanism of action for idiosyncratic reactions is not understood; however, it is suspected to be genetically related (Tatro et al., 1986). Therefore, having a close family member who had severe side effects from a particular drug should sound alarm bells, and the patient should be very closely monitored if the drug is to be prescribed.

PREDISPOSING FACTORS.   Not all individuals who ingest a particular drug will exhibit psychiatric symptoms. This suggests that certain factors predispose development of a substance-induced psychotic disorder. Research has shown that genetic factors coupled with the stress of drug use can trigger a functional disorder. Suspected predisposing factors in drug-induced psychotic disorders are

- genetics (e.g., a family history of psychiatric disorders)
- personal history of functional disorder
- physical illness, especially an illness that affects brain tissue (Gilderman, 1979) and
- individuals with a history of substance abuse (Taylor, 1990)

MECHANISMS OF DRUG-INDUCED PSYCHOSES.   Exact drug mechanisms responsible for inducing psychotic behavior are becoming better understood.

The most reasonable hypothesis indicates that raised CNS dopamine (DA) levels cause psychotic behavior (for example, flight from reality, hallucinations, delusions, breaks between thought and action). As we have indicated, support for the dopamine hypothesis relates to a treatment for Parkinson's disease in which exogenous DA, L-Dopa, is administered. However, one unwanted side effect that sometimes occurs with administration of a dopamine drug is schizophrenic-like behavior. Despite the evidence of dopamine's involvement in psychotic behavior, the dopamine theory is regarded as an oversimplification because very high levels of other neurotransmitters (norepinephrine, for example) can also cause psychotic behavior. Although other neurotransmitters and processes are important in the development of psychosis, increases in the amount or binding capacity of dopamine clearly account for many psychotic symptoms.

DRUGS WITH ANTICHOLINERGIC PROPERTIES THAT CAN PRODUCE PSYCHOSIS

Drugs that block the effects of the neurotransmitter acetylcholine (ACh) in the body are described as having **anticholinergic properties** or **side effects**. Anticholinergic effects of drugs can occur from very small doses, especially in children and the elderly. If a patient is experiencing some of the CNS-adverse effects from drug therapy along with physical side effects, it is likely that the aberrant behavior is drug induced.

NON-CNS ANTICHOLINERGIC SIDE EFFECTS.   Non-CNS side effects include decreased sweating, decreased salivation, dry mucous membranes, dilated pupils, facial flushing, tachycardia (increased heart rate), increased blood pressure, decreased bowel activity, and urinary hesitancy or retention (Brown, 1993).

CNS ANTICHOLINERGIC SIDE EFFECTS.   CNS side effects include amnesia, delirium, disorientation, agitation, anxiety, paranoia, restlessness, mania, insomnia, drowsiness, and hallucinations (Brown, 1993). Box 4-2 contains further information on the various types of drugs that may have anticholinergic effects.

ANTI-PARKINSON AGENTS

Parkinson's disease is thought to result from an imbalance between two CNS neurotransmitters, ACh and DA. In this disease, dopaminergic neurons in the substantia nigra are affected, causing a deficit of DA. Because DA and ACh are in opponent process, ACh gets the upper hand. Both exogenous DA and anticholinergics, which hold down ACh, are often prescribed for Parkinson's. An unwanted side effect that sometimes occurs with dopamine drugs is schizophrenia-like behavior.

Box 4-2   Drugs with Anticholinergic Actions

Anti-Parkinson agents have anticholinergic actions. Here are some of the more useful drugs in this category:

Trade Name	Generic Name
Akineton	biperiden
Artane	trihexyphenidyl
Cogentin	benzotropine
Kemadrin	procyclidine
Parsidol	ethopropazine

Antispasmodic drugs are used to treat gastrointestinal problems, including spastic colon, irritable bowel, mucous colitis, and others. This category of drugs includes:

Trade Name	Generic Name
Bentyl	dicyclomine
Donnatal	atropine, scopolamine, hyoscyamine
Levsin	l-hyoscyamine [Olin et al., 1993]

Antipsychotic agents listed previously in Chapter 4 also have anticholinergic actions.

Antihistamines do not all produce the same amount of anticholinergic activity. However, psychotic symptoms are usually only noted with large doses or overdoses.

Tricyclic antidepressants also have anticholinergic actions. For specific drug references, see Chapter 2.

NON-CNS SIDE EFFECTS.   Non-CNS side effects include anorexia, nausea, vomiting, and dry mouth.

CNS SIDE EFFECTS.   CNS side effects include depression with or without suicidal tendencies, hallucinations, delusions, agitation, anxiety, nightmares, euphoria, and dementia.

Representative drugs in this category include:

Trade Name	Generic Name
Larodopa	levodopa
Parlodel	bromocriptine
Sinemet	carbidopa and levodopa
Symmetrel	amantadine (also used to treat the influenza A virus) (Olin et al.,1998)

STIMULANTS

Stimulants are prescribed by doctors for obesity, attention-deficit disorder, and narcolepsy.

NON-CNS SIDE EFFECTS. Non-CNS side effects include dilated pupils, increased heart rate and respiration, blood pressure changes, increased or decreased salivation, tremor, insomnia, and sweating (Maxmen, 1991).

CNS SIDE EFFECTS. CNS side effects include anxiety, agitation, irritability, aggression, confusion, paranoid hallucinations, panic states, and suicidal or homicidal tendencies (Hoffman & Lefkowitz, 1993). The psychotic episodes that can occur with stimulants clinically resembles paranoid schizophrenia behavior.

Amphetamine stimulants include the following:

Trade Name	Generic Name
Dexedrine	dextroamphetamine
Desoxyn	methamphetamine

Nonamphetamine anorexiant agents are appetite suppressors and include the following:

Trade Name	Generic Name
Fastin	phentermine
Ionamin	phentermine
Preludin	phenmetrazine (Olin et al., 1998)

OPIOID ANALGESICS

Opioid analgesics or narcotics are controlled substances that physicians prescribe for moderate to severe pain. Morphine is the prototype of the opioid analgesic class of drugs. Effects of narcotic analgesics are potentiated by the intake of other CNS depressants, including alcohol, BZDs (valiumlike drugs), or other narcotics.

NON-CNS SIDE EFFECTS. Non-CNS side effects include nausea, vomiting, sweating, constipation, abdominal cramps, urinary hesitancy or retention, and decreased blood pressure. These features are most prominent in ambulatory patients who are not experiencing severe pain.

CNS SIDE EFFECTS. CNS side effects include dizziness, sedation, insomnia, anxiety, fear, agitation, euphoria, dysphoria, disorientation, and hallucinations (Olin et al., 1998). Specific opioid analgesics are discussed in Chapter 5.

DIGITALIS GLYCOSIDES

Digitalis glycosides are derived from plants (foxglove or figwort, for example) and are used to treat heart problems.

NON-CNS SIDE EFFECTS.   Non-CNS side effects include anorexia, nausea, vomiting, diarrhea, and cardiac arrhythmias.

CNS SIDE EFFECTS.   CNS side effects include disorientation, confusion, delirium, fatigue, headaches, aphasia, distraction, bizarre thoughts, paranoid delusions, and hallucinations. The best-known drug in this category is Digoxin (lanoxin; Olin et al., 1998).

CORTICOSTEROIDS

Corticosteroids are used systemically to treat endocrine disorders, rheumatic disorders, collagen diseases, dermatologic diseases, gastrointestinal disorders, nervous system disorders (multiple sclerosis), some cancers, and allergic states (Olin et al., 1998).

NON-CNS SIDE EFFECTS.   Non-CNS side effects include fluid retention, weight gain, increased appetite, impaired wound healing, menstrual irregularities, and **hirsutism** (coarsening of body hair).

CNS SIDE EFFECTS.   CNS side effects include steroid psychosis, which is characterized by paranoid ideations, hallucinations, and a clouded sensorium. Other symptoms noted with steroid use are mood swings (including euphoria or severe depression, for example), personality changes, and insomnia. Onset of symptoms usually occurs within 15 to 30 days of drug use. The occurrence of steroid psychosis does not correlate significantly with a history of psychiatric disorders; rather, the incidence of this disorder is dose related. Of patients treated with prednisone at a daily dose of 40 mg or less, 1.3% experienced steroid psychosis, whereas at a daily dose of prednisone of 80 mg or more, 4.6% of the patients developed psychosis. Symptoms remit with dose reductions, and antipsychotic medications can be used to control these symptoms when steroid therapy cannot be discontinued or the dose cannot be greatly reduced.

Only the systemic steroids or drugs that can be administered orally are listed as follows:

Trade Name	Generic Name
Aristocort	triamcinolone
Delta-Cortef	prednisolone
Deltasone	prednisone
Medrol	methylprednisolone
Orasone	prednisone (Olin et al., 1998)

ANABOLIC STEROIDS

Anabolic steroids are closely related to the male hormone androgen and are popular among athletes and body builders because they increase aggressiveness and muscle mass, decrease muscle recovery time after exercise, and decrease healing time after muscle injury. Despite their widespread use, anabolic steroids have only a few approved therapeutic uses, including anemia, some forms of breast cancer, and for hereditary angioedema (Olin et al., 1998).

NON-CNS SIDE EFFECTS.   Non-CNS side effects include acne, nausea, vomiting, and yellowing of eyes and skin. Additional side effects among women include menstrual irregularities, deepening and hoarseness of the voice, male pattern baldness, and hirsutism (abnormal hair growth). In males, additional side effects include early balding and development of enlarged breasts (Olin et al., 1998).

CNS SIDE EFFECTS.   CNS side effects include depression, insomnia, excitation (Olin et al., 1998), mania, and psychosis (Abramowicz, 1990).

CNS DEPRESSANTS

Psychotic behavior can occur during treatment with CNS depressants or during withdrawal from CNS depressants. However, problems are more likely to arise when the sedative-hypnotic or depressant drug is discontinued. The two main categories of CNS depressants are barbiturates and benzodiazepines. Both classes of drugs have been prescribed for sleep problems and anxiety states. For specific drugs in both classes, refer to the listings in Chapter 4.

NON-CNS SIDE EFFECTS.   Non-CNS side effects include a delirium tremenslike syndrome that appears upon withdrawal.

CNS SIDE EFFECTS.   CNS side effects include rage, hostility, paranoia, hallucinations, depression, insomnia, and nightmares (Abramowicz, 1990).

BETA-ADRENERGIC BLOCKING AGENTS

Beta-adrenergic blocking agents (beta blockers) are a group of structurally related compounds used to treat hypertension, migraines, and a variety of heart problems (Olin et al., 1998). A variety of problems can occur, even with a standard dose (Abramowicz, 1990).

NON-CNS SIDE EFFECTS.   Non-CNS side effects include dry mouth, nausea, vomiting, headaches, and lethargy.

CNS SIDE EFFECTS.   CNS side effects include depression, confusion, nightmares, insomnia, dizziness, anxiety, hallucinations, and paranoia.

Beta blockers include the drugs listed here:

Trade Name	Generic Name
Blocadren	timolol
Brevibloc	esmolol
Cartrol	carteolol
Corgard	nadolol
Inderal	propranolol
Kerlone	betaxolol
Levatol	penbutolol
Lopressor	metoprolol
Normodyne	labetalol
Tenormin	atenolol
Sectral	acebutolol
Visken	pindolol (Olin et al., 1998)

DRUG-INDUCED DEPRESSION

Short-term symptoms of a drug-induced depression are indistinguishable from those of a primary or endogenous depression. However, some chronic physical illnesses or genetic factors predispose an individual to a drug-induced depression. Even though depression is frequently noted in individuals who take CNS depressants, it should not be assumed that the CNS depressant is the primary cause of the depression (Swonger & Matejski, 1991).

Drugs That Can Produce Depression

Hypertensives.   An antihypertensive agent prevents or controls high blood pressure. Common drugs in this category include:

Trade Name	Generic Name
Aldomet	methyldopa
Catapres	clonidine
Inderal	propanolol
Ismelin	guanethidine
Lopressor	metoprolol
Minipress	prazosin
Serpasil	reserpine (Fuller & Underwood, 1989)

Reserpine, an older antihypertensive agent, is contraindicated in patients with a history of affective disorders because depression occurs in a significant number of people who use it (7–20%). Reserpine-induced depression can persist for several months after the drug is discontinued, and the depression may be severe enough to end in suicide (Olin et al., 1998).

Oral contraceptives.   The incidence of depression in females taking birth control pills ranges between 5 and 30%. A history of depression appears to be a predisposing factor. Excessive progestin is thought to cause depression. Discontinuation of the oral contraceptives is the usual treatment for this type of depression (Olin et al., 1998).

WITHDRAWAL FROM STIMULANTS.   It is not uncommon for individuals who have used appetite suppressants chronically to experience depression when the stimulant drug is discontinued. Refer to the drugs listed under stimulants in the previous section for names of drugs in this group.

MISCELLANEOUS DRUGS.   Indocin (Indomethacin) is a nonsteroidal anti-inflammatory agent used in the treatment of certain types of arthritis, bursitis, and gout. Indocin is not only noted for causing depression but may also aggravate other psychiatric disturbances (Olin et al., 1998).

DRUG-INDUCED ORGANIC BRAIN SYNDROME

Approximately 20% of the admissions in psychiatric hospitals are patients diagnosed with **organic brain syndrome (OBS)**. OBS is used to describe an assortment of conditions characterized by impaired brain functioning without indicating the etiology of the impairment (Swonger & Matejski, 1991). CNS impairment in OBS interferes with one or more of the following brain processes: recent or remote memory, orientation, consciousness, intellect, insight, judgment, thought content (hallucinations or illusions), or mood (Thomas, 1985).

Many different types of OBS have been identified. OBS can be reversible (acute) or irreversible (chronic). Dementia and delirium are two global forms of OBS. **Dementia** refers to the loss of intellectual ability that results in impairment in occupational and social functioning. About 20% of dementias are reversible, and this statistic needs to be communicated to patients' families. Alzheimer's disease is an example of an irreversible, degenerative dementia that is not drug induced. **Delirium** is a state of clouded consciousness, in which an individual is unable to focus or sustain attention. Perceptual disturbances, hallucinations and illusions, sleep and affective disturbances, disorientation, and memory impairment are all components of delirium (APA, 1994).

Other types of OBS with specific etiologies have been identified, including, for example, *amnesic syndrome* (e.g., Wernicke-Korsakoff), which results from vitamin B1 deficiency seen in alcoholism (Swonger & Matejski, 1991).

Numerous mechanisms are responsible for producing organic brain syndrome symptoms, including certain drug therapies and interactions of a drug with a medical disorder, fever, infections, inflammatory conditions, brain lesions, and brain tumors. Although some drugs act directly on CNS tissue and alter its functioning, others are indirect, including:

- inadequate brain oxygen caused by decreased cerebral blood flow due to a reduction in cardiac output or blood pressure and
- decreased brain glucose use resulting from low blood sugar (Taylor, 1990)

DRUGS THAT CAN CAUSE OBS

A variety of drugs can cause organic brain syndrome, including drugs that cause hypotension, diuretics, hypoglycemic agents, drugs with anticholinergic properties, and sedative-hypnotics.

DRUGS THAT CAUSE HYPOTENSION.   Many drugs and categories of drugs have hypotensive properties, the ability to reduce blood pressure. Significant reductions in blood pressure may lead to obvious confusion and disorientation. Geriatric patients are especially vulnerable to the hypotensive effects of drugs. Classes of drugs with hypotensive properties include antihypertensives, antipsychotics, tricyclic antidepressants, monoamine oxidase inhibitors, and narcotics (Swonger & Matejski, 1991).

DIURETICS.   A diuretic is a drug that increases the amount of urine excreted by the kidney. Mental functioning can be impaired by overdiuresis or excessive fluid and electrolyte loss. The confusion, lethargy, dizziness, and anxiety caused by diuretics can be reversed by discontinuing the agents and correcting the fluid and electrolyte abnormalities (Swonger & Matejski, 1991). Individuals with eating disorders often abuse diuretics to achieve higher weight loss; thus, their electrolyte balance needs to be closely monitored during treatment.

HYPOGLYCEMIC AGENTS.   Hypoglycemic agents are drugs that have the ability to lower the blood sugar level in the body. Reductions in blood sugar caused by dosage errors in insulin and oral hypoglycemics can be so drastic that bizarre behavior, slurred speech, irrational fear, delusions, hallucinations, and mental confusion may occur (Taylor, 1990).

DRUGS WITH ANTICHOLINERGIC PROPERTIES.   Besides having the potential for inducing psychotic behavior, drugs with anticholinergic properties may also precipitate a state of delirium. This unwanted confusional state is more likely to occur in the geriatric population. Therefore, anticholinergic agents should be prescribed with caution to the elderly (Taylor, 1990).

SEDATIVE-HYPNOTIC DRUGS.   Geriatric patients and individuals with preexisting organic problems are especially vulnerable to the sedative effects of hypnotics, tranquilizers, anxiolytics, antipsychotics, tricyclic antidepressants, and antihistamines. For this reason, conservative use of these medications is recommended in these susceptible populations (Swonger & Matejski, 1991).

CHAPTER 4 REVIEW QUESTIONS

1. What are the primary characteristics of psychotic behavior and how are chronic psychotic states usually subdivided?

2. Under what conditions are antipsychotic medications appropriate?
3. List the five most important demographics associated with individuals with schizophrenia—for example, numbers, spread, mortality, concurrent recreational drug use, etc.
4. How is schizophrenia distinguished from other psychoses according to DSM-IV criteria and what are its major subtypes?
5. Define positive and negative features of schizophrenia and describe the etiology and treatment of each.
6. What is the dopamine hypothesis of schizophrenia?
7. Define and identify implications of the stress diathesis model of mental illness.
8. What are the conditions that should alert therapists that a client may be moving into a relapse?
9. List five ways in which depression affects the remission and exacerbation of schizophrenia and other psychoses.
10. What role does psychotherapy play in the concurrent treatment of schizophrenia?
11. What accounts for the therapeutic effects of the neuroleptics and other antipsychotics?
12. What are extrapyramidal side effects and how are they explained?
13. Describe differences between traditional and new generation antipsychotic medications?
14. What is a psychotoxic drug?
15. What have been some of the consequences of deinstitutionalizing large numbers of patients with schizophrenia over the last 30 years?

WEB RESOURCES ABOUT SCHIZOPHRENIA

In your Internet browser, either Netscape or Internet Explorer, there is a blank space available where you can type the following URL addresses. URL addresses are universal resource locations that start with the letters "http://" and show you a page of information on the Internet. Type any of the following URL addresses into that space and press return in order to go to that page. A variety of access buttons (highlighted words that you may point and click on) are available for further information.

Please note that because of the continuously changing sites, we cannot guarantee that pages will remain at their location address. If pages are incomplete, use the address without the last part of the extension (instead of using http://www.schizophrenia.com/newsletter/, use http://www.schizophrenia.com)

A. http://www.schizophrenia.com/newsletter/newpages/consumer.html
What information does this URL address provide?
This page lists the causes, diagnosis, treatment, and medications involved in schizophrenia (for example, the brain chemistry behind schizophrenia and

the treatments of work therapy and medications like Haldol and Mellaril). Personal stories from person's experiencing schizophrenia and support groups are listed. Each topic includes reviews from the latest research ensuring new information. These, among other related topics, are included, as well as other URL locations on the Internet where one can find information.

How can this page be used?

The left of the screen provides the variety of broad topics relating to schizophrenia. To find out information about that topic, select the topic by clicking on its name. Upon selecting the topic, general information and other specific topics about the topic is presented. For example, upon selecting "What Causes Schizophrenia?" another page is presented identifying a general idea about the cause and then other topics. Topics available will continually change based on updated information.

The bottom of the screen contains a list of topics. To go to the introductory page of this address, you may select "home." To find information out through the newsletter of this site's organization, you may select "news." To chat and discuss information with other persons on the Internet who are interested in this topic, you may select "Family/Consumer Discussion Area".

B. http://www.nmha.org/info/factsheets/51.html

C. http://schizophrenia.nami.org/schizophrenia/schizophrenia.html

D. http://www.mentalhealth.com/fr20.html

5

Pain and the Analgesics

The experience of pain involves both an awareness of an uncomfortable sensation and an emotional reaction to the hurting episode. Pain is much more than a sensory experience; it is an emotional experience that can have lasting effects on the psyche. The emotional and sensory components of pain are mediated through different centers in the brain (Melzack, 1986). The cognitive representations of the hurting episodes, the anticipation of how the discomfort will affect the future, and the emotional background and immediate "surround" all have an impact on the experience of pain. It is for these reasons, and because clients taking pain medications are often seen in psychotherapy, that we have included pain medications.

Chronic back pain, the most expensive single pain complaint, is an excellent example of an acute injury that often leads to psychological referral for a chronically painful condition. Altmaier and Johnson (1992) provide the following summary:

- Eighty percent of adults will have significant low back pain, and about 30% of them will seek medical attention. Of this medical use group, 35% will be pain free in 1 month, 70% pain free in 2 months, 86% pain free in 3 months, and 96% pain free in 1 year.
- The approximately 3% who are disabled include 75,000 workers.
- The total expense for all back injuries in health care costs, disability payments, lost work, and lawsuits totaled $60 billion in 1977, and 25% of the injury cases accounted for around 87% of the total costs.

133

The overall expenditure of $1 for therapy among this medical group saves approximately $3 in future medical costs. Unfortunately, psychotherapy and rehabilitation counseling (by a trained rehabilitation therapist as opposed to a hospital worker with rehabilitation experience) is too often seen as a last resort rather than as an ordinary complement to physical rehabilitation.

UNDERSTANDING THE CHARACTERISTICS OF PAIN

Pain is considered useful in that it is an informative process responsible for alerting the body to a harmful condition. It is, therefore, an adaptive mechanism. In the disease model, treatment of pain focuses on removal of the underlying cause (Berntzen & Gotestam, 1987). However, intensive medical and surgical approaches often fail to uncover the etiology of pain. This is often the case with **chronic pain**, which lasts longer than 3 months and is often not directly associated with continuing tissue damage (Supernaw, 1991a). Chronic pain resulting from progressive malignancies, neuropathies, arthritic conditions, and other states have identifiable sources and are frequently treated more aggressively than chronic pain without a known etiology. Supernaw (1991a) indicates that **acute pain** usually lasts less than 30 days and is deemed functional.

Chronic pain frequently originates as an acute episode then evolves into a prolonged condition. Unfortunately, treatment attempts such as multiple surgeries (and the numerous narcotic prescriptions that accompany them) often exacerbate chronic pain states by adding further injury, scar tissue, and nerve damage to the original site. The majority of chronic pain conditions persist for years in contrast with the short-lived placebo effects of some medications. After numerous treatment attempts, chronic pain sufferers are suspected of not experiencing "real pain"—even though their pain is the product of physical insult—and psychotherapy is belatedly recommended.

Pain without specific etiology or background insult is frequently labeled psychogenic (Fordyce & Steger, 1979). Physicians sometimes confuse psychogenic pain and chronic pain, assuming that an injury that has "healed" should no longer cause pain unless that pain produces some secondary gain. Why pain continues to be produced in old injury sites is not completely clear. Pain specialists have found, however, that the nerves that send pain impulses are sensitized in such a way that they continue to send higher levels of impulses than are warranted by the healing injury.

Berntzen and Gotestam (1987) make a similar distinction between types of pain but employ different terms. *Respondent pain* follows tissue damage, whereas *operant pain* may or may not result from tissue damage. Another distinguishing factor is that the behavior involved in operant pain may be reinforced by either social attention or by reduction of tension, fear, or anxiety. Most pain includes both respondent and operant events. The psychological and emotional consequences of chronic pain are often experienced as suffering—feelings of hopelessness, despair, and anxiety—all of which reflect the subjective experience of pain (Fordyce & Steger, 1979).

Physical pain with a purely psychogenic origin is rare. Physical pain that continues chronically after an acute injury episode is over is very common. Injury to the body through stress-related factors and their painful aftermath (tension headache, for example), is also quite common. Psychological problems cause physical problems that cause pain and exacerbate pain from injuries. The mind, however, rarely creates pain out of whole cloth, without an underlying physical referent.

In the same way that doctors and other health care workers often underestimate their patients' unwillingness to adopt better health care practices (for example, quitting smoking), they often overestimate the ability of patients to resolve chronic pain conditions without psychological help and without the onus that they, by virtue of some psychological dysfunction, are causing the pain to continue long after it should have stopped. Blaming the victim magnifies patient problems and makes it more difficult to treat the psychological component of their pain reaction and attendant suffering.

It should be emphasized that most patients with chronic pain who are successfully treated psychologically do not reduce their pain levels to a major degree. They do come to terms with their physical problem, however, and are more likely to have developed better emotional coping strategies and better *mental* health. It is likely that successful psychological treatment accounts for no more than 20% of the variance in the experience of pain; the other 80% is the result of dimensions of the pain experience that we simply do not understand at this point in our medical knowledge and over which we have much too little control.

Diagnosis of the etiology and ramifications of present pain is of crucial importance in later treatment. Patients who have been told or led to believe that their pain is all in their head make very difficult clients, not only because this view is false in a vast majority of cases but also because it undermines trust in the therapeutic relationship by blaming the patient.

PAIN PATHWAYS

To understand how analgesics work, you must be acquainted with the body's pain pathways. Pain receptors in the skin are referred to as **nociceptors**. When nociceptors are stimulated with noxious stimuli, messages are sent to the spinal cord where the neurotransmitter substance P is released. Substance P sends the pain messages to brain centers by way of two neural pain pathways. These two ascending pain pathways are responsible for the sensory component during a painful experience, whereas the pain's emotional aspect is mediated by the limbic system (Carlson, 1991; Julien, 1996).

The body also has built-in mechanisms to combat the sensation of pain. Two descending inhibitory pain (or analgesic) pathways have been identified. One analgesic pathway originates in the locus ceruleus (located in the medulla of the brain). Activation of this pathway causes the release of the neurotransmitter NE in the spinal cord. NE acts to inhibit the release of substance P, thereby producing an analgesic effect. The brain's second natural analgesic pathway begins in the midbrain and medulla, ultimately affecting delivery of serotonin in the spinal cord. In the spinal cord, serotonin triggers the release of endogenous opioids, which in turn inhibit liberation of substance P. Considering the mechanisms involved in the two descending inhibitory pain pathways, drugs that increase the body's serotonin or potentiate NE (antidepressants, for example) have analgesic effects (Julien, 1996).

A MULTIDISCIPLINARY APPROACH TO TREATMENT

In an effort to obtain relief, chronic pain patients tend to overutilize the medical system (Deardoff, Rubin, & Scott, 1991). Berntzen and Gotestam (1987) contend that pain behavior is positively reinforced by pain medications, and, thus, help-seeking behavior may be prolonged. Whether or not the pain behavior is reinforced, it is clear that chronic, low-level pain does not respond well to management with morphine or its synthetic derivatives, and tolerance to and dependence on them grow very rapidly. Unfortunately, drug therapy for chronic, nonlifethreatening pain leads all too often to abuse and dependence.

Chronic pain is maintained by multiple factors. Therefore multidisciplinary rather than unidimensional treatment is recommended. Prototypical multidisciplinary pain programs involve active physical therapy, stress and anxiety management, body mechanics and posture training, relaxation and self-regulating procedures, biofeedback, pain medication reduction, and individual or group therapy (Deardoff et al., 1991). Deardoff et al. (1991) conducted a study comparing the effects of a comprehensive multidisciplinary treatment program for a group of chronic pain patients with a group who received no treatment. Results showed that the multidisciplinary approach was more effective in producing increased physical functioning, decreased drug use, and an increase in the return-to-work rate. The no treatment group did not experience similar improvements. Importantly, however, there was little difference between the two groups in their subjective experiences of pain. Therefore, the primary goal of multidisciplinary pain programs is to increase functioning and return to normalcy—that is, *reduction of suffering*. Pain reduction (reduction of pain perception) is an important but secondary goal. Clearly, pain perception should not and does not always lead to subjective suffering!

Tension headaches cause chronic pain for many individuals. Supernaw (1991b) recommends behavior modification, eliminating tension-causing ingredients such as caffeine from the diet, and investigating the possible precipitating roles anxiety and depression may play in the occurrence of tension headaches. Other underlying psychiatric problems (and, importantly, physiological processes like temporal mandibular joint (TMJ) problems, for example) may also be at work and should be investigated if behavioral techniques do not provide incremental relief.

STRATEGIES FOR DELIVERY OF ANALGESICS

Counselors may work with clients who are in severe or progressive pain situations. In these circumstances, new strategies for delivery of analgesics and dosing schedules are useful, and we will include them in this discussion.

Physicians frequently prescribe pain medications on a PRN basis. **PRN** means *pro re nata* or that medications are given on demand or as needed (Berntzen & Gotestam, 1987). Yet PRN analgesic administration is problematic. With chronic pain sufferers as subjects, Berntzen and Gotestam (1987) conducted a study comparing the effects of PRN (pain-contingent) dosing with fixed interval (time-contingent) dosing. Results indicate that a fixed interval schedule is more effective in controlling pain and improving mood. Further, fixed interval dosing regimens are believed to have a lower potential for drug dependence.

Supernaw (1991a) indicates that in severe pain, PRN dosing allows the pain to return before redosing is initiated and that therefore more drug may be used with PRN dosing regimens. Furthermore, employing a regular or fixed administration schedule of pain medication prevents the occurrence of pain memory. Once the pain reappears, the patient begins to anticipate pain distress, which can increase the emotional reaction and elevate the experience of pain.

Patient-controlled analgesia (PCA) is a well-accepted pain management technique. As the name implies, patients control the frequency of the analgesic administration. Usually used in hospital settings, PCA devices consist of a pump that is activated by the patient to initiate infusion of small doses of narcotics into an intravenous catheter. The safety of PCA from overdose is ensured by a built-in mechanism or system of constraints. Drug concentration levels in the blood fluctuate minimally with PCA administration devices, therefore the peak sedative effects do not occur as often (Bedder, Soifer, & Mulhall, 1991). An added psychological benefit with PCA devices is that the patient is empowered by helping combat an adverse experience. Sometimes PCA devices are set to deliver a continuous low dose of pain medication that may be supplemented by patient activation of the device to deliver small supplemental boluses of the same medication; again, built-in constraints along with direct nursing supervision prevent the patient from exceeding a therapeutic level of medication.

Transdermal systems (skin patches) are also being used to administer pain medication for chronic pain conditions. Fentanyl, a narcotic analgesic, is available in this form and is usually effective for 48–72 hours, eliminating the need to frequently readminister the drug to control the pain (Olin et al., 1998).

In treating a variety of medical conditions such as hypertension, physicians routinely begin with a low dosage and then increase it until the desired effect is achieved. Yet, in severe acute pain situations, an aggressive dosing philosophy called *descending the ladder* is recommended. With this dosing method, the starting dose is slightly tapered downward until the patient's pain threshold is discovered. The advantage to this type of dosing philosophy is that the patient's pain is relieved rapidly rather than gradually. The speedy removal of discomfort helps lower the patient's anxiety or emotional reaction, thereby helping to alleviate the experience of pain (Supernaw, 1991a). When a patient's dose of narcotics must be increased to maintain pain relief, as sometimes occurs with progressive malignancies, the sedative side effects of the narcotic may be combatted with amphetamine stimulants or methylphenidate (Ritalin).

HEADACHE PAIN

Of all the recurrent medical conditions, headaches are the most common and the most annoying. A variety of chronic or recurrent headache types are described in the literature. Health care workers note that the *tension headache* (also referred to as *stress, muscle contraction*, or *ordinary* headache) produces the most frequent complaints and plagues 10–20% of the population. Without any warning signs, tension headaches begin with gradual dull and nagging pain affecting both sides of the head (Supernaw, 1991b).

Although not as common as the tension type, *migraine headaches* receive the most attention. Often preceded by a prodromal sign such as blurred vision, a migraine is a vascular headache that produces intense pain lasting 4 to 12 hours. It is caused by dilation of cranial vessels and may put pressure on optic nerves. Most of the time, migraine pain occurs on only one side of the head. Patients may also experience nausea, vomiting, and diarrhea. Hypersensitivity to lights or sound often occurs with migraines. Additionally, physical exertion has been shown to aggravate them. A genetic component may be involved, for migraines are known to run in families (Supernaw, 1991b).

Some of the agents used in the treatment and prevention of migraine headaches have not been mentioned yet. An ergot alkaloid drug (ergotamine) causes constriction of cranial blood vessels and is valuable in aborting and preventing migraines. Because ergot alkaloids are toxic drugs, they should only be taken as prescribed by a physician. A related drug, methysergide, is used only as a prophylactic for migraine or vascular headaches. Two other agents, timolol and propanolol, are also helpful in preventing migraines. These two drugs are members of a group of drugs called *beta blockers*, which are better known for their cardiovascular effects. Finally, drugs that raise levels of 5-HT successfully treat many migraine sufferers. Sumatriptan (Imitrex), as well as the heterocyclic AMs, are becoming more widely used.

CHRONIC PAIN IN THE ELDERLY

Chronic pain is common in the elderly because of the high prevalence of arthritis, cancer, and vascular disease in this population, yet analgesic prescription and drug use declines with advancing age. The reasons for this reduction are not clear. Nevertheless, because of specific factors associated with aging, such as reduced liver and kidney functioning, reduced body mass, and gastric atrophy, the elderly have an increased risk for analgesic toxicity.

TREATMENT WITH NARCOTICS

A notable feature of an analgesic state is that it can occur without a loss of consciousness (Jaffe & Martin, 1985). Analgesic agents, drugs that reduce sensitivity to pain, can be globally categorized into narcotics or non-narcotics. In severe acute or chronic pain with a known etiology, narcotics are frequently prescribed.

Other terms used to refer to narcotic analgesics are **opioids** or **opiates**. Opioids are naturally occurring (endogenous or exogenous) or synthetic drugs that mimic the effects of morphine. Morphine or other similar drugs are extracted from the opium poppy. Dating back to ancient cultures, opium has been used for a variety of different reasons, including both medicinal and recreational purposes. Endogenous opioids, those produced in the body and brain to aid in pain relief, are grouped into three distinct categories: enkephalins, endorphins, and dynorphins. Like their endogenous counter- parts, morphine and morphinelike drugs collectively have a wide range of (mostly) inhibitory effects.

The targeted therapeutic or primary effect of narcotics is analgesia. However, these drugs have been associated with a variety of secondary pharmacological effects or side effects. The most frequently noted side effects are as follows:

System	Effects
CNS	Euphoria, drowsiness, apathy, mental confusion
Gastrointestinal	Constipation, nausea, vomiting
Cardiovascular	Hypotension (decrease in blood pressure) that may produce lightheadedness and fainting
Other	Urinary retention

The most hazardous side effect is respiratory depression, which is dose depen- dent. Respiratory depression can be potentiated by other CNS depressants and may be fatal (Olin et al., 1998).

MECHANISMS OF ACTION

Chemical structures of morphine or synthetic narcotic agents closely resemble the chemical structures of the endogenous opioids, internal neuromodulators

Table 5-1   Opioid Receptors and Their Effects

Receptor	Location	Effects
Mu	Supraspinal (thalamus, brain stem areas including locus caeruleus)	Analgesia, euphoria, respiratory depression, physical depression
Kappa	Spinal cord	Analgesia, sedation, miosis (pin-point pupils)
Sigma	Limbic system	Dysphoria, psychotomimetic effects (such as hallucination)
Delta	Limbic system	Possible mood effect

Sources: Carlson, 1991; Julien, 1992; Olin et al., 1993.

whose main duty is alleviation of physical and mental pain. This resemblance accounts for the narcotic drugs' stimulation of opioid receptors and the concomitant production of an analgesic state. A variety of opioid analgesics exist, but not every opioid drug produces all possible effects. Opioid analgesics differ in their molecular shape and their ability to stimulate specific opioid receptors (Jaffe & Martin, 1993).

Five major categories of opioid receptors have been identified; they are *mu, kappa, sigma, delta,* and *epsilon*. Table 5-1 lists the opioid receptors along with the usual effects of their stimulation.

Opioid drugs exert their principal effects by activating CNS opioid receptors located in the spinal cord, the brain stem, and the limbic system. The analgesic effect of opioids involve not only an alteration in sensation of pain but changes in affective responses to the pain. The action of several different systems of neurotransmitters (for example, norepinephrine and serotonin effects on substance P) are components of the analgesic effects of narcotics (Jaffe & Martin, 1993).

CLASSIFICATION OF NARCOTIC ANALGESICS

Opioid drugs are classified as agonists, antagonists (or pure antagonists), or mixed agonist–antagonists.

NARCOTIC AGONISTS

If a drug stimulates an opioid receptor, producing morphinelike actions, the drug is referred to as an agonist. Narcotic agonists activate mu receptors and, to a lesser extent, activate the kappa and sigma opioid receptors (Julien, 1996). Some narcotic agonists are naturally occurring compounds (for example, morphine and codeine); others are synthetic or semisynthetic drugs. Table 5-2 lists the more popular narcotic agonists.

Table 5-2   Narcotic Agonists

Trade Name	Generic Name	Other Information
Codeine	codeine	Also used as a cough suppressant
Darvon	propoxyphene	In excessive doses has been asso- ciated with drug-related deaths
Demerol	meperidine	
Dilaudid	hydromorphone	
Dolophine	methadone	Also used in detoxification programs
Duragesic	fentanyl	Transdermal system skin patch worn for 72 hours
Levo-Dromoran	levorphanol	
MS Contin	morphine	A controlled release tablet
Opium Tincture	paregoric	Mostly used as an antidiarrhea drug
Roxanol	morphine	
Roxicodone	oxycodone	

Note: Drugs available only in injectable or suppository form are not listed.

Source: Olin et al., 1993.

In the 1800s, Brompton's Mixture was used as a pain cocktail for people suffering from progressive pain such as that associated with cancer. It was an amalgamation of morphine, cocaine, chloroform, and alcohol. Today's pain cocktail usually contains only morphine and is often referred to as a Hospice Mixture (Supernaw, 1991a). Sometimes other ingredients, such as aspirin, Tylenol, tricyclic antidepressants, antihistamines, or stimulants may be included (Olin et al., 1998).

To decrease the dose of narcotic agents or to increase the effectiveness of less potent analgesics, it is common for Tylenol (acetaminophen) or aspirin to be combined with a narcotic. It is important to be aware of narcotic analgesic combinations because of their potential for abuse and depressive effects. Table 5-3 lists narcotic analgesic combinations that are frequently prescribed.

NARCOTIC ANTAGONISTS

Narcotic antagonist drugs can bind with opioid receptors but do not produce analgesic activity. These agents block the effects of narcotic agonists and can precipitate withdrawal in narcotic drug-dependent individuals. Obviously, narcotic antagonists are not used as analgesics. Table 5-4 lists the two drugs in this grouping, along with their uses.

MIXED AGONIST–ANTAGONIST ANALGESICS

Mixed agonist–antagonist drugs can stimulate some opioid receptors while blocking others. Most of these agents have an affinity for activating sigma

Table 5-3   Frequently Prescribed Narcotic Analgesic Combinations

Trade Name	Components
Darvocet-N 50	propoxyphene 50 mg/acetaminophen 325 mg
Darvocet-N 100	propoxyphene 100 mg/acetaminophen 650 mg
Darvon-N w/ASA	propoxyphene 100 mg/aspirin 325 mg
Darvon Compound	propoxyphene 32 mg/aspirin 389 mg/caffeine 32.4 mg
Darvon Compound 65	propoxyphene 65 mg/aspirin 389 mg/caffeine 32.4 mg
Empirin/Cod #2	codeine 15 mg/aspirin 325 mg
Empirin/Cod #3	codeine 30 mg/aspirin 325 mg
Empirin/Cod #4	codeine 60 mg/aspirin 325 mg
Fiorinal/Cod #3	codeine 30 mg/acetaminophen 325 mg/caffeine 40 mg/ butalbital 50 mg
Lortab	hydrocodone 2.5 mg
Lortab 5	hydrocodone 5 mg/acetaminophen 500 mg
Lortab 7	hydrocodone 7.5 mg/acetaminophen 500 mg
Mepergan Fortis	meperidine 50 mg/promethazine 25 mg
Percodan	oxycodone 5 mg/aspirin 325 mg
Percocet	oxycodone 5 mg/acetaminophen 325 mg
Phenaphen/Cod #2	codeine 15 mg/acetaminophen 325 mg
Phenaphen/Cod #3	codeine 30 mg/acetaminophen 325 mg
Phenaphen 650/Cod	codeine 30 mg/acetaminophen 650 mg
Phenaphen/Cod #4	codeine 60 mg/acetaminophen 325 mg
Synalgos-DC	dihydrocodeine 16 mg/aspirin 356.4 mg
Tylenol/Cod #1	codeine 7.5 mg/acetaminophen 300 mg
Tylenol/Cod #2	codeine 15 mg/acetaminophen 300 mg
Tylenol/Cod #3	codeine 30 mg/acetaminophen 300 mg
Tylenol/Cod #4	codeine 60 mg/acetaminophen 300 mg
Tylox	oxycodone 5 mg/acetaminophen 500 mg
Wygesic	propoxyphene 65 mg/acetaminophen 650 mg

Source: Olin et al., 1993.

receptors, which can result in dysphoric and hallucinogenic experiences (Julien, 1996). An advantage this group of narcotic analgesics has is that it has a lower potential for abuse (Olin et al., 1998). Also, Supernaw (1991a) purports that these agents produce less respiratory depression. However, they are not

Table 5-4   Narcotic Antagonists and Their Uses

Trade Name	Generic Name	Use
Narcan	naloxane drug	Treat narcotic overdoses
Trexan	naltrexone	Help maintain an opioid-free state in detoxified opioid-dependent individuals

Source: Olin et al., 1993.

recommended in progressive pain situations because of their low therapeutic dose ceiling. The agonist–antagonist drugs are:

Trade Name	Generic Name
Stadol NS	butorphanol
Talwin	pentazocine

OTHER ANALGESICS

SALICYLATE ANALGESICS

Aspirin, the most famous salicylate analgesic, was introduced in 1899 (Insel, 1993). Besides being effective in treating mild to moderate pain, it is an effective agent in inflammatory processes, including tissue damage and arthriticlike conditions. Aspirin is also valued for its antipyretic (fever reducing) action. Because aspirin inhibits blood platelet aggregation, lengthening blood clotting time, it is useful in preventing myocardial infarctions (heart attack).

Aspirin's analgesic activity is attributed to its effect on inhibiting prostaglandin synthesis. Being highly bound to proteins in the blood, aspirin's potential for interactions with other drugs is considerable. Gastrointestinal (GI) problems such as nausea, anorexia, and GI bleeding are the most frequent side effects associated with aspirin use. For this reason, it is recommended that aspirin be taken with food (Olin et al., 1998). However, because aspirin and acetaminophen decrease prostaglandins that work to protect the stomach and intestinal wall, both can cause stomach problems even when not absorbed through the stomach. Aspirin has the advantage over narcotic analgesics of being a nonaddictive agent. The average dose of aspirin will vary with the condition for which it is prescribed or indicated; however a common adult dose is one to two tablets (325 mg each) every 4 hours as needed. The usual adult dose is provided as a basis for comparison with the approximate acute lethal dose for adults, which is 10,000 mg to 30,000 mg (approximate lethal dose for children is 4000 mg). Ear problems, such as dizziness or tinnitus (ringing in the ears), are early warning signs of aspirin toxicity (Olin et al., 1998).

ACETAMINOPHEN

Tylenol (acetaminophen) is a viable alternative for individuals who should not take aspirin. It is equipotent to aspirin's analgesic and antipyretic effects. However, acetaminophen is void of anti-inflammatory properties, so its scope of usefulness is less than that of aspirin.

Acetaminophen's mechanism of action for its analgesic effect is not completely clear, but acetaminophen, like aspirin, inhibits prostaglandin synthesis in the CNS. However, in the peripheral nervous system, its ability to inhibit prostaglandin synthesis is minimal (Olin et al., 1998). Because it is metabolized in the liver, acetaminophen should be used with caution in individuals with liver problems. Severe liver damage has resulted from using normal therapeutic doses of acetaminophen while drinking. Further, it has been reported that chronic use of high doses of acetaminophen (5000 mg or more per day, approximately ten extra-strength tablets) for 2 to 3 weeks have resulted in extensive liver damage and even death (Supernaw, 1991a).

NONSTEROIDAL ANTI-INFLAMMATORY DRUGS (NSAIDs)

NSAIDs are widely used, and the selection of a specific agent is determined by the physician and the nature of the problem. Although not more effective than aspirin, NSAIDs are recommended when pain is nonresponsive to aspirin therapy (Supernaw, 1991a). Egbert (1991) claims that the analgesic activity of NSAIDs is similar to that of weak narcotic analgesics such as propoxyphene (Darvon). NSAIDs possess anti-inflammatory, antipyretic, and analgesic activity. The exact mode of action is not known, but their ability to inhibit prostaglandin synthesis is important. Similar to aspirin, the major drawback of NSAID usage is GI problems. Also, these drugs are highly protein-bound, so the potential for drug interactions is significant. Drowsiness, dizziness, and blurred vision are included in NSAIDs' side effects. Therefore, when taking NSAIDs, consumption of alcohol is contraindicated (Olin et al., 1998).

Many drugs are included in this category. Among the various agents, differences exist not only in the duration of action, frequency of dosing, and side effects but also in the efficacy in treating a variety of conditions. Table 5-5 lists the most common NSAIDs.

ADJUNCTIVE ANALGESIC TREATMENTS

Another type of medication offers promise as an adjunct to analgesics. Utilizing tricyclic and heterocyclic (second generation) antidepressants as supplemental medication in chronic pain conditions appears to be beneficial. These antidepressant analgesic effects operate by inhibiting the reuptake of the

Table 5-5   Nonsteroidal Anti-Inflammatory Drugs (NSAIDs)

Trade Name	Generic Name	Trade Name	Generic Name
Advil	ibuprofen	Nalfon	fenoprofen
Anaprox	naproxen	Naprosyn	naproxen
Ansaid	flurbiprofen	Orudis	ketoprofen
Clinoril	sulindac	Ponstel	mefenamic acid
Feldene	piroxicam	Relafen	nabumetone
Indocin	indomethacin	Telectin	tolmetin
Lodine	etodolac	Toradol	ketorolac
Meclomen	meclofenamate	Voltaren	diclofenac
Motrin	ibuprofen		

neurotransmitters serotonin and norepinephrine. Increased serotonergic activity is associated with a rise in the pain threshold, while lowered serotonergic activity lowers the pain threshold (Trimble, 1990).

Chronic pain conditions for which antidepressants may be useful are migraine headaches, chronic tension headaches, diabetic neuropathy, tic douloureux, cancer pain, peripheral neuropathy with pain, post-therapeutic neuralgia, fibromyalgia, and arthritic pain. Tricyclics that may be prescribed for chronic pain include but are not limited to the following:

Trade Name	Generic Name	Dose
Adapin	doxepin	50–300 mg per day
Elavil	amitriptyline	50–100 mg per day
Endep	amitriptyline	50–100 mg per day
Sinequan	doxepin	50–300 mg per day
Tofranil	imipramine	75–150 mg per day
		(Olin et al., 1993)

Drugs prescribed for migraine headaches include the following:

Trade Name	Generic Name
Blocadren	timolol
Ergostat	ergotamine (a sublingual tablet)
Inderal	propanolol
Medihaler Ergotamine	ergotamine (an inhaler)
Sansert	methysergide
	(Olin et al., 1993)

NARCOTIC ABUSE AND TOXICITY

A characteristic feature of all opioid narcotic drugs is their potential for drug tolerance, psychological and physical dependence, and addiction. Because of the propensity for narcotic use to transform into drug abuse, these drugs are carefully monitored by the U.S. Drug Enforcement Administration (DEA). By providing stringent guidelines to pharmaceutical companies, doctors, nurses, and pharmacists, the DEA closely monitors distribution, dispensing, and administration of these drugs.

Unfortunately, illicit narcotic usage patterns are common. In the scope of their practices, physicians and pharmacists are liable to ensure that abusive patterns of narcotic usage do not develop. Situations of abuse often evolve when patients are under the care of more than one doctor, creating a situation where physicians are unaware of the drugs other doctors prescribe for their patients. If the patient patronizes only one drugstore and that store maintains a patient profile system, the pharmacist can easily detect excessive narcotic prescribing. However, the patient may be using many different pharmacies. This action makes it difficult for the attending druggists and the doctors to collect accurate information on the amount of narcotics the patient has been prescribed. It is imperative, therefore, that counselors gather as much information as possible about drug prescriptions and drug intake. Measures to create statewide and national databases that monitor prescription drug use have been resisted politically under the umbrella of the right to privacy.

Warnings associated with narcotic use are numerous. The dangerous depressant effects of opioid drugs are potentiated by the intake of other CNS depressants such as alcohol, barbiturates, benzodiazepines, or other sedative-hypnotic agents. The possibilities for lethal combinations of narcotics with other depressants are abundant. In such cases, the cause of death is usually respiratory depression and failure. Signs of opioid toxicity include respiratory depression, extreme somnolence, skeletal muscle flaccidity, and cold clammy skin (Olin et al., 1998). Opioid antagonists (Narcan, for example) have an excellent record for reversing the effects of narcotics overdose. Those suspected of narcotics overdose should be viewed as medical emergencies.

CHAPTER 5 REVIEW QUESTIONS

1. What are some factors that influence the experience of pain?
2. What is the most expensive single pain complaint and why? Statistically, what is the impact of therapy?
3. When is chronic pain likely to be treated less aggressively?
4. What physiological explanation may account for pain that continues after tissue healing has occurred?
5. How do most chronic pain patients who have undergone psychological treatment benefit from the experience?
6. Why is a multidisciplinary approach to pain management often advocated? What are some of the typical components?
7. What are the benefits of fixed interval dosing of pain medication?
8. Why are tricyclic antidepressants analgesic?
9. What is an opioid agonist? Antagonist?
10. What is substance P and what other neurotransmitters interact with it to modulate its importance?
11. What are potential difficulties in using aspirin, acetaminophen, and NSAIDs?

WEB RESOURCES ABOUT CHRONIC PAIN

In your Internet browser, either Netscape or Internet Explorer, there is a blank space available where you can type the following URL addresses. URL addresses are universal resource locations that start with the letters "http://," and show you a page of information on the Internet. Type any of the following URL addresses into that space and press return in order to go to that page. A variety of access buttons (highlighted words that you may point and click on) are available for further information.

Please note that because of the continuously changing sites, we cannot guarantee that pages will remain at their location address. If pages are incomplete, use the address without the last part of the extension (instead of using http://www.cdc.gov/ncidod/diseases/cfs/cfshome.htm, use http://www.cdc.gov/).

A. http://www.cfids.org/

What information does this URL provide?

Chronic fatigue and immune dysfunction syndrome, symptoms (such as visual disturbances, chills, and night sweats), and treatments (such as dietary restrictions and medications) are discussed. This page also gives information about the latest chronic fatigue research, news and support groups available, and information about how to receive disability benefits.

How can this page be used?

In the middle of the page several buttons are available that, when pointed to and clicked on, will provide further information. Some of the buttons are as follows:

About the Association	CFIDS Research
Understanding CFIDS	Disability
News and Advocacy	The CFIDS Chronicle

Click on the button "Understanding CFIDS" and other buttons will appear such as "What are other common symptoms?," "How is CFIDS treated?," and several other topics. When clicking on one of these buttons, further information regarding that topic will appear on the screen.

B. http://www.cdc.gov/ncidod/diseases/cfs/cfshome.htm

C. http://www.sunflower.org/~cfsdays/cfsfiles.htm

D. http://www.cais.com/cfs-news/

WEB RESOURCES ABOUT HEADACHE PAIN

In your Internet browser, either Netscape or Internet Explorer, there is a blank space available where you can type the following URL addresses. URL addresses are universal resource locations that start with the letters "http://" and show you a page of information on the Internet. Type any of the following URL addresses into that space and press return in order to go to that page. A variety of access buttons (highlighted words that you may point and click on) are available for further information.

Please note that because of the continuously changing sites, we cannot guarantee that pages will remain at their location address. If pages are incomplete, use the address without the last part of the extension (instead of using http://www.ama-assn.org/insight/spec_con/migraine/migraine.htm, use http://www.ama-assn.org/insight/spec_con/migraine/.)

A.   http://www.ama-assn.org/insight/spec_con/migraine/migraine.htm
What information does this URL address provide?

This page provides information on similarities and differences among various types of headaches (such as migraine, cluster, and tension-type headaches). Causes and symptoms of headaches, nondrug treatments (such as biofeedback, relaxation training, and cognitive-behavioral therapy) and drug treatments (such as nonprescription analgesics, acetaminophen combined with a sedative, and antidepressants) are discussed. This page also gives information on how to find a doctor and other types of support.

How can this page be used?

In the middle of the page a variety of topics are presented. Topics in bold color, such as "Headache Types and Their Treatments," and "Important Information About Drugs That Prevent Migraine," can be clicked on for further information. For example, click on "How is Migraine Treated?" and another page will appear with two more buttons: "Targeting 'Provokers' of Migraine" and "Migraine Management." These can be clicked on for further information.

On the left of the page, the topics "Family Focus," "Hospital Select," and "Physician Select," when clicked, show information provided by the American Medical Association (AMA) on how to assist the family, how to select a physician, and other information.

On the bottom of the page in black, topics are presented that can be clicked on to locate information on the AMA site, such as "Medical and Science Education," "Advocacy and Communications," and "Links."

B. http://www.migrainehelp.com/

C. http://www.excedrin.com/

D. http://www.headaches.org/topics.html

WEB RESOURCES ABOUT FIBROMYALGIA

In your Internet browser, either Netscape or Internet Explorer, there is a blank space available where you can type the following URL addresses. URL addresses are universal resource locations that start with the letters "http://" and show you a page of information on the Internet. Type any of the following URL addresses into that space and press return in order to go to that page. A variety of access buttons (highlighted words that you may point and click on) are available for further information.

Please note that because of the continuously changing sites, we cannot guarantee that pages will remain at their location address. If pages are incomplete, use the address without the last part of the extension (instead of using http://www.arthritis.ca/frames/types.html, use http://www.arthritis.ca/).

A. http://www.arthritis.ca/frames/types.html
What information does this URL address provide?

This page lists information (diagnosis, symptoms, treatment, prognosis, etc.) for several different types of arthritis (fibromyalgia, osteoarthritis, reactive arthritis, etc). The page also makes available various treatment and coping information, support groups and bibliotherapy, statistical information, and an open forum for discussing fibromyalgia and other types of arthritis.

How can this page be used?

On the left of the screen, categories of information are presented. To find information within a category, click on the phrase. For example, the "Living Well with Arthritis" category, when pressed, makes available a page with different topics, such as "Family Issues," "Exercise," "Pain Management," and "Communicating Your Needs." Other categories, such as "Programs and Resources," "The Politics of Arthritis," and "Research in Action," when clicked, will also provide further topics and detailed information.

On the middle of the page, a white rectangular box appears with "Types of Arthritis" and various types of arthritis will be listed. Select a type by clicking on it. For example, point and click on "Fibromyalgia." The list will disappear and "Fibromyalgia" will appear in the box where "Types of Arthritis" was located. Now that you have selected the type, press the "Submit" box. Another page appears listing topics to be addressed regarding fibromyalgia. Click on the topic (for example, Diagnosis, Treatment, or Prognosis) and detailed information will appear about that topic.

B. http://members.aol.com/fibroworld/

C. http://www.fmagw.org/

D. http://www.teleport.com/~nfra/Guide.htm#Top

APPENDIX A

THE NERVOUS SYSTEM

Hundreds of years of research and thousands of volumes of literature have been devoted to explaining the structure and function of the human nervous system. For the purpose of this text, a simple outline is offered to familiarize the reader with this very complex system that controls our physical movements, thoughts, and emotional reactions. The nervous system consists of two major divisions. The central nervous system (CNS) includes the brain and spinal cord. The peripheral nervous system (PNS) consists of all the nervous tissue outside the CNS. Throughout the nervous system, there are two basic cell types, neurons and glial cells. Recall that the interaction of neurons is what causes our behaviors.

THE CENTRAL NERVOUS SYSTEM (CNS)

The numerous physical structures that comprise the central nervous system are amazing and their relationships to each other are highly complex. The brief mentioning of only a few parts of this remarkable system and its organization seems remiss. However, only a few of the important CNS structures or systems are explained. One of the CNS's protective barriers is a three-layered covering called the *meninges*. The meninges encapsulates both of the CNS's two major divisions, the spinal cord and the brain (Carlson, 1991). Infection of this protective barrier is the dreaded, lifethreatening condition known as meningitis.

Other important brain structures include the cerebral cortex, the hypothalamus, the thalamus, the cerebellum, the reticular formation, the pons, and the medulla.

The cerebral cortex is the outer layer of the forebrain and is the most sophisticated and recent evolutionary development of the brain. It is often called the "gray matter" because the numerous cell bodies in this area have a grayish-brown appearance. Under the gray matter lie millions of myelinated axons that have a white appearance, and this area is called the "white matter." (Axons are extensions of neurons.)

The cerebral cortex is divided front to back into the right and left hemispheres. Most people have heard information on the brain's hemispheres and that the right brain hemisphere controls the left side of our bodies and that the left brain hemisphere controls the right side of our bodies. The *corpus callosum* is the main group of axons or nerve tissue that connects the right hemisphere with the left hemisphere. Each cerebral hemisphere has four areas or lobes, and each lobe has a specific function:

- frontal lobe—planning and movement
- parietal lobe—sensory stimulation
- occipital lobe—vision
- temporal lobe—hearing and memory

The *hypothalamus* is a collection of nuclei, which are groups of neuron cell bodies located inside the CNS. The hypothalamus controls the autonomic nervous system (ANS) and the endocrine system and organizes survival behavior (fighting, feeding, fleeing, and mating) for the species. The hypothalamus produces hormones that travel to the nearby anterior pituitary gland. This gland is referred to as the body's "master gland" because it controls other glandular secretions, such as sex and growth hormones. The hypothalamic hormones stimulate secretion of hormones from the anterior pituitary gland.

The *thalamus* is a large two-lobed structure located in the center of the brain. The thalamus receives information from sensory systems and relays messages to various areas in the brain. The thalamus is informally referred to as the "Grand Central Station" of the CNS.

The *cerebellum* is a distinct brain structure that is connected to the back of the brain stem. The cerebellum functions in coordination of movement, maintenance of equilibrium, and regulation of muscle tone. Drugs (alcohol, for example) that slow down activity in the cerebellum may lead to disequilibrium, loss of motor control, and, at very high or toxic levels, death.

The *reticular formation* is a structure in the core of the brain stem. It is important for controlling alertness, waking, sleeping, muscle tone, and various reflexes. The *pons* is a part of the brain stem and includes part of the reticular formation. The pons plays an important role in sleep and arousal. The *medulla* (or medulla oblongata) is also a component of the brain stem. It controls vital functions such as regulating the cardiovascular system, regulating respiration and skeletal muscle tone and is located at the top of the spinal cord.

SYSTEMS THAT ENCOMPASS NUMEROUS AREAS OF THE BRAIN

The organization of the brain also includes subsystems, which involve various brain structures in controlling specific functions. An important brain subsystem is the *reticular activating system* (RAS), which extends from the central core of the brain stem to the cortex. The RAS is essential in initiating and maintaining wakefulness, introspection, and directing attention. Various tranquilizing drugs (benzodiazepines such as Valium, for example) suppress the RAS. Several stimulant drugs, such as amphetamines, activate the RAS. Continuous stimulation or intermittent overstimulation can lead to a wide range of psychiatric difficulties, including anxiety, paranoia, and panic.

Another important subsytem in the human brain are the pyramidal tracts. *Pyramidal tracts* are the main motor neuron tracts of the body. They originate in the cerebral cortex and cross over in the medulla. These nerve tracts are responsible for conducting the motor impulses from one side of the brain to the skeletal muscles on the opposite side of the body.

Extrapyramidal tracts, much more complex than pyramidal tracts, function to conduct impulses needed for muscle tone and equilibrium. Drugs that are said to produce extrapyramidal symptoms usually impair fine muscle coordination and balance and produce stereotypic, repetitive facial, tongue, and hand muscle twitches. Unfortunately, common side effects of the older antipsychotic medication produce these unwanted motor movements.

The *brain stem*, another brain subsystem, is located at the base of the brain or the top of the spinal cord. The brain stem has three basic functions: (a) to relay messages to and from the cerebrum, cerebellum, and spinal cord; (b) to act as a component in various CNS activities such as the sleep–wake cycle, consciousness, and respiratory and cardiovascular control; and (c) to facilitate activities of the cranial nerves. Most of the 12 cranial nerves' cell bodies originate in the brain stem. Three prominent CNS structures, the medulla, the pons, and the midbrain, make up the brain stem.

The *limbic system* is a group of interconnected structures located underneath the cerebral cortex. Some of the important structures within this important brain subsystem are the amygdala and hippocampus. The limbic system also connects to the hypothalamus and septal area of the brain. The limbic system is active in motivation, emotions, mood, and in other processes. This system is the site of action of many drugs that alter moods and feeling states.

THE PERIPHERAL NERVOUS SYSTEM

Communication between the CNS (brain and spinal cord) and the rest of the body is accomplished via spinal nerves and cranial nerves. The peripheral nervous system (PNS) is comprised of all the nervous tissue outside the CNS, including the 12 cranial nerves and 31 spinal nerves.

Cranial nerves consist of 12 pairs of nerves that mostly serve the sensory and motor functions in the head and neck region. Special names are given to each pair of nerves, with the name of the nerve suggesting its function.

Spinal nerves are the collection of 31 nerve pairs that branch out from the front and back of the spinal cord. No special names are assigned to the spinal nerves. Each set of nerves is represented by a number that corresponds to the level of the spinal column on which the nerve pair originates. There are 8 cervical, 12 thoracic, 5 lumbar, 5 sacral pairs, and 1 coccygeal pair of spinal nerves. Nerve fibers that carry messages or commands from the spinal cord to organs, muscles, or glands are called *efferent fibers* or axons. Sensory information that is perceived is relayed to the spinal cord along *afferent fibers* or axons.

The PNS is made up of two major divisions. The somatic nervous system receives information from sensory neurons and controls skeletal movement. The autonomic nervous system (ANS) is sometimes referred to as the involuntary nervous system. The ANS functions to regulate smooth muscle, cardiac muscle, and glands; it governs actions of various organ systems (stomach, pancreas, intestines, lungs, bladder, sweat glands, salivary glands, skin, sex organs, and more). ANS has two main divisions, the **parasympathetic nervous system** and the **sympathetic nervous system**. Both systems innervate nerves to most organs. The parasympathetic nervous system controls "feed and breed" activities during times of relaxation, producing a decrease in heart rate and an increase in digestive activity. The parasympathetic system also facilitates activities that increase the body's supply of stored energy. The sympathetic nervous system is activated in times of excitement and exertion known to produce the body's "fight or flight" responses. It mobilizes energy, increases blood flow to vital skeletal muscles, stimulates the release of adrenalin, and increases heart rate and the level of sugar in the blood. Highly anxious individuals are likely to have an active sympathetic nervous system.

GLOSSARY

Acetylcholine (ACh)   One of the major neurotransmitters, located both in the central and peripheral nervous systems. ACh plays an excitatory role in processes involving memory, mood, learning, attention, muscular contraction, and sleep.

Action potential (AP)   A change in a nerve's electrical charge to the extent that the nerve is stimulated.

Acute pain   Pain, due to disease or injury, that lasts less than 30 days and that is functional in restricting movement of the person or injured area.

Adrenalin   A neural transmitter produced by the adrenal gland, exerting most of its effect in the peripheral nervous system where it functions to maintain heart rate and blood pressure. Also referred to as *epinephrine*.

Agonist   A drug or chemical that increases the availability for action or mimics the action of an endogenous neurotransmitter.

Akathisia   A physical state of nervousness that is characterized by compulsion to move or in which an individual is in constant motion. This conditon is often characterized as "restless legs," fidgetiness, and agitation.

Akinesia   A complete or partial loss of muscular movement.

Amino acids   A group of organic compounds used as the building blocks of proteins. Some also act as neurotransmitters.

Antagonist   A drug that decreases the availability or action of a neurotransmitter.

Anticholinergic properties   The properties of drugs that block the action of the neurotransmitter acetylcholine. Side effects include dry mouth, constipation, blurred near vision, urinary retention, increased heart rate, and delayed ejaculation.

Anxiolytic   An agent that reduces anxiety. Also referred to as a *minor tranquilizer*.

Ataxia   Lack of muscular coordination.

Autonomic nervous system (ANS)   A branch of the nervous system that is concerned with involuntary control in the body. The ANS has two major divisions, the parasympathetic nervous system and the sympathetic nervous system.

Axon   Part of a neuron—generally shaped like a long, slender tube—that relays impulses from the soma (cell body of the neuron) to the terminal buttons of the neuron.

Barbiturates   A class of central nervous system–depressant drugs that were once frequently prescribed as sedatives.

155

Benzodiazepines (BDZs) A group of structurally related compounds that have sedative properties. Because of their greater safety margin, BDZs have, for the most part, replaced the barbiturates, a more dangerous class of sedatives.

Beta blockers or beta-adrenergic blocking agents A group of structurally related drugs used to treat hypertension, migraines, a variety of heart problems, and other problems.

Biological amine hypothesis of depression The view that functional deficits in the brain of the catecholamine NT norepinephrine or the indoleamine NT serotonin—or both—cause depression.

Blood-brain barrier (BBB) A barrier in the central nervous system that exists between circulating blood in the brain and the fluid that surrounds the brain tissue.

Bruxism Teeth grinding while sleeping.

Catecholamines A class of neurotransmitters derived from the compound catechol. Each neurotransmitter in this group has an amine group. Neurotransmitters in this class are dopamine, norepinephrine, and epinephrine.

Chronic pain Pain that evolves into a prolonged or long-term episodic condition of more than 3 months and that can no longer be directly attributed to continuing tissue damage.

Convergence of information The gathering of information from many other neurons by dendrites.

Delirium A state of clouded consciousness in which an individual is unable to focus or sustain attention. Perceptual disturbances (hallucination and illusions), sleep and affective disturbances, disorientation, and memory impairment are all components of delirium.

Delta waves The deep restorative sleep in the human sleep cycle.

Dementia A loss of intellectual ability that results in impairment in occupational and social functioning.

Dendrite A part of the neuron that branches off toward other nerve cells. Dendrites contain receptors, which receive messages from other nerve cells.

Depolarization A process that occurs when a neuron becomes more positive, producing an excitatory effect. Also referred to as *excitatory postsynaptic potential (EPSP)*.

Diuretic An agent that increases the amount of urine the kidney excretes.

Divergence of information The dispersal of information by axons to many other neurons.

Dopamine (DA) A neurotransmitter that produces both excitatory and inhibitory effects in the central nervous system. Dopamine is involved in movement, learning and attention, Parkinson's disease, and schizophrenia.

Dopamine hypothesis of schizophrenia The view that either functional changes in the catecholamine NT dopamine in the brain or an excess of dopamine causes schizophrenia.

Double depression A state that occurs when individuals with dysthymia also experience an episode of major depression.

Drug allergy A situation wherein any amount of a particular drug introduced into the body elicits an allergic response.

Drug holiday A period of time when a routinely prescribed drug is deliberately not administered.

Dynorphins An endogenous group of opioid neurotransmitters that have analgesic effects.

Dyskinesia   Side effects of antipsychotic drugs. Dyskinesia is characterized as inappropriate movements (spasms, tics, and involuntary movements).

Dyssomnias   A group of sleep disorders with the chief problem being amount, quality, or timing of sleep.

Dysthymia   Depressive neurosis marked by either long-term depression or chronic, but subacute, depression.

Dystonic reactions   Side effects of antipsychotic drugs. Dystonic reactions are characterized by involuntary and inappropriate postures.

Electroencephalogram (EEG)   The polygraphic recording of the brain's electrical activity (brain waves).

Endocytosis   The process through which neurotransmitters are reuptaken.

Endorphins   Endogenous neurotransmitters that have an analgesic effect similar to morphine. Also referred to as *opioid peptides.*

Enkephalins   An endogenous group of opioid neurotransmitters with analgesic effects.

Enzymatic deactivation   A degradation process of a neurotransmitter by an enzyme.

Enzyme   Organic compounds in living cells. Enzymes act as catalysts for a variety of the body's chemical reactions.

Enzyme induction   The process by which the liver is induced to manufacture higher levels of enzymes to break down either naturally occurring body chemicals or exogenous drugs.

Epinephrine (Epi)   A neurotransmitter produced by the adrenal gland. Epinephrine exerts most of its effect in the peripheral nervous system, where it functions to maintain heart rate and blood pressure. Also referred to as *adrenalin.*

Excitatory postsynaptic potential (EPSP)   A process that occurs when a neuron becomes more positive, producing an excitatory effect. Also referred to as *depolarization.*

Exocytosis   The process of a neuron releasing neurotransmitters into the synapse.

Extrapyramidal symptoms   A group of side effects commonly associated with antipsychotic medications. Extrapyramidal symptoms include Parkinsonian symptoms, dystonic reaction, tardive dyskinesia, dyskinesia, and akathisia.

Functional disorder   A general term applied to a condition when reasons for change in function are not apparent.

Functional psychoses   Abnormal behaviors that cannot be attributed to any single known cause.

Galactorrhea   Abnormal flow of breast milk or lactation.

Gamma-aminobutyric acid (GABA)   An inhibitory neurotransmitter found in the brain.

Glial cells   Support cells, found in the nervous system, that function in various ways.

Glutamate   An excitatory neurotransmitter that lowers the threshold for neural excitation.

Glycine   A neurotransmitter that has inhibitory effects in the spinal cord.

Gynecomastia   A condition of abnormally large mammary glands in males (milk may be secreted).

Half-life   The average time required to eliminate one-half of a drug's dose.

Heterocyclic antidepressants   A broad class of antidepressant drugs developed and introduced after tricyclic antidepressants; often called *second generation antidepressants.*

Hirsutism   Abnormal hair growth.

Hyperpolarization   A process whereby a neuron's electrical charge becomes more negative, causing an inhibitory or stabilizing effect on the neuron. Also called *inhibitory postsynaptic potential (IPSP)*.

Hypnotic   A drug capable of inducing a state of central nervous system depression that resembles normal sleep.

Hypoglycemic agent   A drug with the ability to lower the body's blood sugar level.

Hypomania   A state of mild mania and excitement with modest behavioral change.

Idiosyncratic reaction   A side effect that occurs in only a very small percentage of the population.

Inhibitory postsynaptic potential (IPSP)   A process whereby a neuron's electrical charge becomes more negative, causing an inhibitory or stabilizing effect on the neuron. Also called *hyperpolarization*.

Insomnia   A perceived decrease in the quality or quantity of sleep, which affects the individual's daytime functioning.

Ions   Small, electrically charged molecules.

Lipid   A fat or fatlike substance.

Lipophilic molecules   Molecules that dissolve readily in fats. *Lipophilic* is a term used to describe a substance's (or drug's) affinity for fats.

Lysergic acid diethylamide (LSD)   A psychedelic drug that is similar in structure to the neurotransmitter serotonin.

Major tranquilizer   Another term for antipsychotic drugs.

Meninges   A three-layered covering that encapsulates the central nervous system (brain and spinal cord).

Minor tranquilizer   An agent that reduces anxiety. Also referred to as an *anxiolytic*.

Monoamine oxidase inhibitor antidepressants (MAOIs)   A group of antidepressant agents that exert their desired effect by inhibiting the enzyme monoamine oxidase, which is normally responsible for the degradation of monoamine neurotransmitters.

Monoamines   A class of neurotransmitters. Each neurotransmitter in this group has a single amine group as part of its chemical structure. Neurotransmitters in this class include dopamine, norepinephrine, epinephrine, and serotonin.

Myelin sheath   A protective covering of axons. The myelin sheath also improves distance conduction.

Narcolepsy   A sleep disorder characterized by excessive daytime sleepiness, falling asleep at inappropriate times, cataplexy, sleep paralysis, and hypnogogic hallucinations.

Neuralgia   A condition of severe, sharp nerve pain.

Neuroleptic   Phenothiazine drugs and Haldol. Neuroleptics are used to treat the positive symptoms of schizophrenia.

Neuroleptic malignant syndrome   A very severe, potentially lifethreatening complication that can occur when using antipsychotic drugs. The syndrome is characterized by catatonia, unstable blood pressure, unstable heart rate, hyperthermia, mutism, muscle rigidity, and stupor. When this condition is left untreated, the mortality rate is nearly 30%.

Neuroleptic state   A state induced in

schizophrenics when treated with antipsychotic drugs. A neuroleptic state is characterized by psychomotor slowing, emotional quieting, and affective indifference.

Neuromodulators (NMs)   Chemicals that facilitate communication between neurons.

Neuron   A highly specialized nerve cell that conducts impulses throughout the brain and body.

Neuropeptides   Chains of amino acids that either act on their own or act to enhance or inhibit the effects of other neurotransmitters.

Neuropharmacology   The study of drugs' effects on the nervous system.

Neurotransmission   Communication between neurons.

Neurotransmitters (NTs)   Chemicals that facilitate communication between neurons.

Nightmares   Dreams with anxiety-provoking content. Nightmares are often open to recall and occur during REM sleep.

Night terrors   A sleep disorder characterized by extreme vocalizations, sweating, or fast heart rate.

Nociceptor   A pain receptor located in the skin.

Norepinephrine (NE)   An excitatory neurotransmitter involved with emotions and with maintaining wakefulness and alertness.

Opiate   A naturally occurring or synthetic analgesic agent that mimics the effects of morphine.

Opioid peptides   Endogenous neuropeptide analgesic agents. Also referred to as *endorphins*.

Opioids   Another term for opiates or narcotic analgesics.

Opponent process   A situation in which excitatory and inhibitory neurotrans-

mitter systems counteract each other to have a balancing effect.

Organic brain syndrome   A term used to describe an assortment of conditions characterized by impaired brain functioning without indicating the etiology of the impairment.

Organic psychoses   Psychotic behavior that results from insult or trauma to the brain.

Parasomnias   A group of sleep disorders characterized by an abnormal event during sleep.

Parasympathetic nervous system   A division of the autonomic nervous system that is active during times of relaxation.

Parkinsonian effects or symptoms   Side effects that resemble symptoms of Parkinson's disease. They are common in antipsychotic drug therapy.

Parkinson's disease   A chronic progressive disease characterized by rigidity, tremors, and muscle weakness resulting from an imbalance of dopamine and acetylcholine in the brain.

Pharmacokinetics   The study of in vivo drug processes, including administration, absorption, distribution, metabolism, and excretion.

Pharmacopsychologist   A psychologist trained as an expert in psychoactive medications who may or may not have prescription privileges.

Pharmacopsychology   The study of psychoactive medications. Also referred to as *psychopharmacology*.

Phenothiazines   The oldest class of antipsychotic drugs. All have a similar chemical structure.

Polydipsia   Excessive thirst.

Polypharmacy   Condition of being treated with an excessive number of prescription drugs.

Polyuria   Excessive urination.

PRN   In drug therapy, PRN (*pro re nata*) refers to medication given on demand or as needed.

Prophylactic treatment   Drug therapy used to prevent the onset or recurrence of a disease.

Protein binding   The ability of a drug to attach to proteins circulating in the bloodstream.

Psychotoxic   Drugs that alter central nervous system functioning. Also referred to as *psychotropic*.

Psychotropic   Drugs that alter central nervous system functioning. Also referred to as *psychotoxic*.

Rapid eye movement (REM) sleep   One of the sleep stages; characterized by regular, fast eye movements; muscle paralysis; and occurrence of dream activity.

Rebound hyperexcitability   A state of rapid rise of neural excitation due to abrupt discontinuation of tranquilizing drugs.

Receptor   Specialized molecules on neurons that are targets for specific neurotransmitters.

Reuptake   The process of extremely rapid removal of the neurotransmitter from the synaptic cleft.

Second generation antidepressants   A group of newer antidepressants that are less toxic and have fewer side effects than the older tricyclic antidepressants.

Serotonin (5-HT)   A neurotransmitter involved in the inhibition of activity and behavior. It is active in mood regulation; control of eating, sleeping, and arousal; and pain regulation.

Signal anxieties   Anxieties that signal (result from) unresolved psychodynamic conflicts and that usually do not remit until underlying issues are resolved.

Sleep apnea   A sleep disorder characterized by cessations in breathing interfering with the quality of sleep.

Soma   The cell body of the neuron. The soma holds the nucleus and gives rise to the axon.

Somatic nervous system   One of the two main divisions of the peripheral nervous system. The somatic nervous system is active in receiving information for sensory neurons and controlling skeletal movement.

Somnambulism   Sleepwalking.

Steroid psychosis   Psychotic behavior precipitated by the use of corticosteroids.

Stress-diathesis model   Stress in the environment interacting with an individual's genetic predisposition to trigger the onset of an illness.

Substance P   A neurotransmitter released in the spinal cord to facilitate relaying pain messages.

Sympathetic nervous system   One of the divisions of the autonomic nervous system that is activated in times of excitement or stress.

Synapse   The point where two neurons meet and relay information.

Synaptic cleft or gap   The area between two adjacent neurons in which neurotransmitters travel.

Tardive dyskinesia   A late-appearing side effect of antipsychotic drugs. Tardive dyskinesia is characterized by abnormal, involuntary movements (tics and tremors) of the mouth, face, limbs, and trunk. This condition is sometimes disfiguring or incapacitating.

Teratogenic effects   Development of a severely abnormal or deformed fetus due to the mother's ingestion of drugs during pregnancy.

Terminal buttons   Knob-like structures, located on the end of a neron's axon, where neurotransmitters are stored.

Therapeutic window   The range in which a drug's doses are both safe and effective. A wide therapeutic window or margin indicates that a drug's therapeutic dose is much lower than its toxic dose.

Tricyclic antidepressants (TCAs)   A class of antidepressants with the same basic three-ring chemical structure. Tricyclic agents are notorious for their bothersome side effects.

Vesicle   A small sac inside a neuron's terminal button that contains the neurotransmitter.

REFERENCES

ABRAMOWICZ, M. (Ed.). (1990, January 16). Drugs that cause psychiatric symptoms. *The Medical Letter, 31,* 113–118.

ALLEBECK, P. (1989). Schizophrenia: A life-shortening disease. *Schizophrenia Bulletin, 15,* 81–89.

ALTMAIER, E. M., & JOHNSON, B. D. (1992). Health-related applications of counseling psychology: Toward health promotion and disease prevention across the life span. In S. Brown & R. Lent (Eds.), *Handbook of counseling psychology* (2nd ed., pp. 315–348). New York: Wiley.

AMERICAN MEDICAL ASSOCIATION. (1983). Antipsychotic drugs. In *AMA drug evaluations*. Philadelphia: Saunders.

AMERICAN PSYCHIATRIC ASSOCIATION. (1994). *Diagnostic and statistical manual of mental disorders* (4th ed.). Washington, DC: American Psychiatric Association.

ANDREASEN, N. C. (1989). The American concept of schizophrenia. *Schizophrenia Bulletin, 15*(4), 519–531.

ANGERMEYER, M. C., KUHN, L., & GOLDSTEIN, J. M. (1990). Gender and the course of schizophrenia: Differences in treated outcomes. *Schizophrenia Bulletin, 16*(2), 293–305.

BALDESSARINI, R. J. (1985). Drugs and the treatment of psychiatric disorders. In A. G. Gilman, L. S. Goodman, T. W. Rall, & F. Murad (Eds.), *The pharmacological basis of therapeutics* (7th ed., pp. 387–445). New York: Macmillan.

BALDESSARINI, R. J. (1993). Drugs and the treatment of psychiatric disorders. In A. G. Gilman, T. W. Rall, A. S. Nies, & P. Taylor (Eds.), *The pharmacological basis of therapeutics* (8th ed., pp. 383–435). New York: McGraw-Hill.

BARLOW, D. H. (1988). *Anxiety and its disorders: The nature and treatment of anxiety and panic*. New York: Guilford Press.

BARLOW, D. H., & CERNY, J. A. (1988). *Psychological treatment of panic*. New York: Guilford Press.

BARON, M., GRUEN, R., RAINER, J. D., KANE, J., ASNIS, L., & LORD, S. (1985). A family study of schizophrenia and normal control probands: Implications for the spectrum concept of schizophrenia. *American Journal of Psychiatry, 142*(4), 447–455.

BEASLEY, C. M., DORNSEIF, B., BOSOMWORTH, J., SAYLER, M., RAMPEY, A., HEILIGENSTEIN, J., THOMPSON, V., MURPHY, D., & MASICA, D. (1991). Fluoxetine and suicide: A meta-analysis of controlled trials of treatment for depression. *BMJ, 303,* 685–692.

BEASLEY, C. M., MASICA, D., & POTVIN, J. (1992). Fluoxetine: A review of receptor and functional effects and their clinical implication. *Psychopharmacology, 107,* 1–10.

BECK, A. T., & EMERY, G. (1985). *Anxiety disorders and phobias: A cognitive perspective*. New York: Basic Books.

BECK, A. T., RUSH, A. J., SHAW, B. F., & EMERY, G. (1979). *The cognitive therapy of depression.* New York: Guilford Press.

BEDDER, M. D., SOIFER, P. E., & MULHALL, J. J. V. (1991). A comparison of patient-controlled analgesia and bolus PRN intravenous morphine in the intensive care environment. *Clinical Journal of Pain, 7*(3), 205–208.

BELLACK, A. S. (1989). A comprehensive model for treatment of schizophrenia. In A. S. Bellack (Ed.), *A clinical guide for the treatment of schizophrenia* (pp. 1–22). New York: Plenum.

BERNTZEN, D., & GOTESTAM, K. G. (1987). Effects of on-demand versus fixed-interval schedule in the treatment of chronic pain with analgesic compounds. *Journal of Consulting and Clinical Psychology, 55*(2), 213–217.

BOSZORMENYI-NAGY, I., & KRASNER, B. R. (1986). Between give and take: A clinical guide to contextual therapy. New York: Brunner/Mazel.

BRANCONNIER, R. J., COLE, J. O., GHAZVINIAN, S., SPERA, K., OXENKRUG, G. F., & BASS, J. L. (1983). Clinical pharmacology of bupropion and imipramine in elderly depressives. *The Journal of Clinical Psychiatry, 44*(5), 130–134.

BRENNER, H. D., DENCKER, S. J., GOLDSTEIN, M. J., HUBBARD, J. W., KEEGAN, D. L., KRUGER, G., KULHANEK, F., LIBERMAN, R. P., MALM, U., & MIDHA, K. K. (1990). Defining treatment refractoriness in schizophrenia. *Schizophrenia Bulletin, 16*(4), 551–561.

BROWN, J. H. (1993). Atropine, scopolamine, and related antimuscarinic drugs. In A. G. Gilman, T. W. Rall, A. S. Nies, & P. Taylor (Eds.), *The pharmacological basis of therapeutics* (8th ed., pp. 150–165). New York: McGraw-Hill.

BROWN, W. A., & HERZ, L. R. (1989). Response to neuroleptic drugs as a device for classifying schizophrenia. *Schizophrenia Bulletin, 15*(1), 123–128.

BUSSE, E., & SIMPSON, D. (1983). Depression and antidepressants and the elderly. *The Journal of Clinical Psychiatry, 44*(5), 35–40.

CASSEM, E. H. (1995). Depressive disorders in the medically ill. *Psychosomatics, 36*(2), S2–S10.

CARLSON, N. R. (1991). *Physiology of behavior* (4th ed.). Boston: Allyn & Bacon.

CAROFF, S. N., & MANN, S. C. (1988). Neuroleptic malignant syndrome. *Psychopharmacology Bulletin, 24*(1), 25–29.

CHAFETZ, M. D., & BUELOW, G. D. (in press). A training model for psychologists with prescription privilege: Clinical pharmacopsychologists. *Professional Psychology: Research and Practice.*

CHARNEY, D. S., HENINGER, G. R., & BREIER, A. (1984). Noradrenergic function in panic anxiety: Effects of yohimbine in healthy subjects and patients with agoraphobia and panic disorder. *Archives of General Psychiatry, 41,* 751–763.

COOPER, J. R., BLOOM, F. E., & ROTH, R. H. (1991). *The biochemical basis of neuropharmacology.* New York: Oxford University Press.

COURSEY, R. D. (1989). Psychotherapy with persons suffering from schizophrenia: The need for a new agenda. *Schizophrenia Bulletin, 15*(3), 349–353.

CROOK, T. H., KUPFER, D. J., HOCH, C. C., & REYNOLDS, C. F. (1987). Treatment of sleep disorders in the elderly. In H. Meltzer (Ed.), *Psychopharmacology: The third generation of progress* (pp. 1159–1165). New York: Raven Press.

DAWKINS, K., & POTTER, W. (1991). Gender differences in pharmacokinetics and pharmacodynamics of psychotropics: Focus on women. *Psychopharmacology Bulletin, 27,* 417–423.

DEARDOFF, W. W., RUBIN, H. S., & SCOTT, D. W. (1991). Comprehensive multidisciplinary treatment of chronic pain: A follow-up study of treated & non-treated groups. *Pain*, *45*, 35–43.

DELGADO, P. L., PRICE, L., MILLER, H., SALOMON, R., LICINIO, J., KRYSTAL, J., HENINGER, G., & CHARNEY, D. (1991). Rapid serotonin depletion as a provocative challenge test for patients with major depression: Relevance to antidepressant action and the neuro-biology of depression. *Psychopharmacology Bulletin*, *27*, 321–330.

DUGAS, J. E. (1987). Panic disorders: Pathophysiology and treatment. *Pharmacy Times*, *53*(11), 120–131.

EGBERT, A. M. (1991). Help for the hurting elderly. *Post Graduate Medicine*, *89*(4), 217–228.

ELLENOR, G. L., & DISHMAN, B. R. (1996). Mood stabilizers: Lithium, carbamazepine, Valproic Acid. In K. Stovell (Ed.), *Psychotropic medication* (pp. 195–198). Providence, Rhode Island: Manisses Communications Group, Inc.

FERRIS, R. M., COOPER, B. R., & MAXWELL, R. A. (1983). Studies of bupropion's mechanism of antidepressant activity. *The Journal of Clinical Psychiatry*, *44*(5), 74–79.

FORDYCE, W. E., & STEGER, J. C. (1979). Chronic pain. In O. F. Pomerleau & J. P. Brady (Eds.), *Behavioral medicine: Theory and practice* (pp. 125–153). Baltimore: Wilkins & Wilkins.

FREDRICK, J. F., & FREDRICK, N. J. (1985). The hospice experience: Possible effects in altering the biochemistry of bereavement. *The Hospice Journal*, *1*(3), 81–90.

FULLER, S. H., & UNDERWOOD, E. S. (1989, August). Update on antidepressant medications. *U.S. Pharmacist*, pp. 35, 36, 39, 42, 44, 46.

GADOW, K. D. (1992). Pediatric psychopharmacotherapy: A review of recent research. *Journal of Child Psychology and Psychiatry*, *33*, 153–195.

GARVEY, M. (1990). Benzodiazepines for panic disorder. *Postgraduate Medicine*, *90*(5), 245–246, 249–252.

GILDERMAN, A. (1979). Drug-induced psychiatric illnesses. In Hoffman-LaRoche, Inc., *Psychopharmacology for practicing pharmacists*. Pamphlet. New Jersey: Nuttley.

GOODNICK, P. J. (1991). Pharmacokinetics of second generation antidepressants: Bupropion. *Psychopharmacology Bulletin*, *27*, 516–519.

GOSSEL, T. A., & WUEST, J. R. (1992). Alzheimer's disease, part 1: Pathogenesis, symptoms and outcome. *Mississippi Pharmacist*, *18*(4), 27–29.

GOVONI, L. E., & HAYES J. E. (1994). *Drugs and nursing implications*. Connecticut: Appleton-Century-Crofts.

GRINSPOON, L. (Ed.). (1994). Sleep disorders—Part II. *The Harvard Mental Letter*, *11*(3), 1–5.

GRINSPOON, L. (Ed.). (1996). How does melatonin affect sleep? *The Harvard Mental Health Letter*, *12*(12), 8.

GUTHRIE, S., BROWN, C., & CYR, M. (1996). Reactions to antidepressants: Cyclics, SSRIs, miscellaneous. In K. Stovell (Ed.), *Psychotropic medications* (pp. 121–122). Providence, Rhode Island: Manisses Communications Group, Inc.

HALL, R. C., & WISE, M. G. (1995). The clinical and financial burdens of mood disorders. *Psychosomatics*, *36*(2), S11–S18.

HAMMEN, C. L. (1991). Mood disorders. In M. Hersen & S. M. Turner (Eds.), *Adult psychopathology and diagnosis* (2nd ed.). New York: Wiley.

HAURI, P. J. (1985). Primary sleep disorders and insomnia. In T. L. Riley (Ed.), *Clinical aspects of sleep and sleep disturbances*. Boston: Butterworth.

HEINRICHS, D. W., & CARPENTER, W. T. (1985). Prospective study of prodromal symptoms in schizophrenic relapse. *American Journal of Psychiatry, 142*(3), 371–373.

HOFFMAN, B. B., & LEFKOWITZ, R. J. (1993). Catecholamines and sympathomimetic drugs. In A. G. Gilman, T. W. Rall, A. S. Nies, & P. Taylor (Eds.), *The pharmacological basis of therapeutics* (8th ed., pp. 221–243). New York: McGraw-Hill.

INSEL, P. A. (1993). Analgesics-antipyretics and anti-inflammatory agents: Drugs employed in the treatment of rheumatoid arthritis and gout. In A. G. Gilman, T. W. Rall, A. S. Nies, & P. Taylor (Eds.), *The pharmacological basis of therapeutics* (8th ed., pp. 638–681). New York: McGraw-Hill.

JAFFE, J. H., & MARTIN, W. R. (1985). Opioid analgesics and antagonists. In A. G. Gilman, L. S. Goodman, T. W. Rall, & F. Murad (Eds.), *The pharmacological basis of therapeutics* (7th ed., pp. 491–531). New York: Macmillan.

JAFFE, J. H., & MARTIN, W. R. (1993). Opioid analgesics and antagonists. In A. G. Gilman, T. W. Rall, A. S. Nies, & P. Taylor (Eds.), *The pharmacological basis of therapeutics* (8th ed., pp. 485–521). New York: McGraw-Hill.

JESTE, D. V., & WYATT, R. J. (1982). *Understanding and treating tardive dyskinesia.* New York: Guilford Press.

JOHNSON, D. A. (1989). Treatment of depression in schizophrenia. In B. Lerer & S. Gershon (Eds.), *New directions in affective disorders* (pp. 509–516). New York: Springer-Verlag.

JONAS, J. M., & SCHAUMBURG, R. (1991). *Everything you need to know about Prozac.* New York: Bantam.

JOYCE, P. R., & PAYKEL, E. S. (1989). Predictors of drug response in depression. *Archives of General Psychiatry, 46*(1), 89–99.

JULIEN, R. M. (1996). *A primer of drug action* (8th ed.). New York: W. H. Freeman.

KANE, J. M. (1989). Innovations in the psychopharmacologic treatment of schizophrenia. In A. S. Bellack (Ed.), *A clinical guide for the treatment of schizophrenia* (pp. 43–76). New York: Plenum.

KIMBERLY, A., ELLISON, J., SHERA, M., PRATT, L., LANGFORD, B., COLE, J., WHITE, K., LAVORI, P., & KELLER, M. (1992). Pharmacotherapy observed in a large prospective longitudinal study on anxiety disorders. *Psychopharmacology Bulletin, 28,* 131–137.

KLAASSEN, C. D. (1993). Nonmetallic environmental toxicants: Air pollutants, solvents and vapors, and pesticides. In A. G. Gilman, T. W. Rall, A. S. Nies, & P. Taylor (Eds.), *The pharmacological basis of therapeutics* (8th ed., pp. 1615–1639). New York: McGraw-Hill.

KLEIN, G. R. (1987). Pharmacotherapy of childhood hyperactivity: An update. In H. Y. Meltzer (Ed.), *Psychopharmacology: The third generation of progress* (pp. 1215–1224). New York: Raven Press.

LAWSON, G. W., & COPPERRIDER, C. A. (1988). *Clinical psychopharmacology.* Gaithersburg, MD: Aspen.

LARCO, J. P., & KODSI, A. B. (1996). Reactions to antipsychotics. In K. Stovell (Ed.), *Psychotropic medications* (pp. 2–3). Providence, Rhode Island: Manisses Communications Group, Inc.

LECCESE, A. P. (1991). *Drugs and society.* Englewood Cliffs, NJ: Prentice Hall.

LICKEY, M. E., & GORDON, B. (1995). *Drugs for mental illness.* New York: Freeman.

LOEBEL, A. D., LIEBERMAN, J. A., ALVIR, J. M., MAYERHOFF, D. I., GEISLER, S. H., & SZYMANSKI, S. R. (1992). Duration of psychosis and outcome in first-episode schizophrenia. *American Journal of Psychiatry, 149*(9), 1183–1188.

MARDER, S. R., MINTZ, J., PUTTEN, T. V., LEBELL, M., WIRSHING, W. C., & JOHNSTON-CRONK, K. (1991). Early prediction of relapse in schizophrenia: An application of receiver operating characteristic (ROC) methods. *Psychopharmacology Bulletin, 27*(1), 79–82.

MAXMEN, J. C. (1991). *Psychotropic drugs fast facts.* New York: Norton.

McBRIDE, P. A., ANDERSON, G., KHAIT, V., SUNDAY, S., & HALMI, K. (1991). Serotonergic responsitivity in eating disorders. *Psychopharmacology Bulletin, 27,* 365–371.

MELZACK, R. (1986). Neurophysiological foundations of pain. In R. A. Sternbach (Ed.), *The psychology of pain* (2nd ed.). New York: Raven Press.

MISHARA, B. L., & KASTENBAUM, R. (1980). *Alcohol and old age.* New York: Grune & Stratton.

MOORCROFT, W. H. (1989). *Sleep, dreaming, and sleep disorders.* Lanham, MD: University Press of America.

MORRIS, G. O., WILLIAMS, H. L., & LUBIN, A. (1960). Misperception and disorientation during sleep deprivation. *Archives of General Psychiatry, 2,* 247–254.

NAPOLIELLO, M. J., & DOMANTAY, A. G. (1991). Buspirone: A worldwide update. *British Journal of Psychiatry, 159,* 40–44.

New Drugs in the Pipeline for Depression, Schizophrenia. (1998, April). *Copy Editor, 9*(4), 1, 6–7.

NOYES, R., CROWE, R. R., HARRIS, E. L., HAMRA, B. J., McCHESNEY, C. M., & CHAUDHRY, D. R. (1986). Relationship between panic disorder and agoraphobia. *Archives of General Psychiatry, 43,* 227–232.

NURSING99 BOOKS. (1999). *Nursing99 Drug Handbook.* Springhouse, PA: Springhouse.

OKUMA, T. (1989). Acute and prophylactic properties of carbamazepine in bipolar affective disorders. In B. Lerer & S. Gershon (Eds.), *New directions in affective disorders* (pp. 535–539). New York: Springer-Verlag.

OLIN, B. R., HEBEL, S. K., DOMBEK, C. E., & KASTRUP, E. K. (Eds.). (1998). *Facts and comparison.* New York: Lippincott.

PARKES, J. D. (1985). *Sleep and its disorders.* Philadelphia: Saunders.

PELHAM, W. E. (1993). Pharmacotherapy with children with attention-deficit hyperactivity disorder. *School Psychology Review, 22,* 199–227.

PLOTKIN, D. A., GERSON, S. C., & JARVIK, L. F. (1987). Antidepressant drug treatment in the elderly. In H. Meltzer (Ed.), *Psychopharmacology: The third generation of progress* (pp. 1149–1158). New York: Raven Press.

PONTEROTTO, J. G. (1985). A counselor's guide to psychopharmacology. *Journal of Counseling and Development, 64,* 109–115.

PRICE, R. H., & LYNN, S. J. (1986). *Abnormal psychology* (2nd ed.). Pacific Grove, CA: Brooks/Cole.

Quetiapine May Be Better Than Others at Treating Aggression. (1998). *Copy Editor, 9*(5), 1, 6–7.

REIMHERR, F. W., CHOUINARD, G., COHN, K., COLE, J., ITIL, T., LAPIERRE, Y., MASCO, H., & MENDELS, J. (1990). Antidepressant efficacy of sertraline: A double-blind, placebo- and amitriptyline-controlled, multicenter comparison study of outpatients with major depression. *Journal of Clinical Psychiatry, 51,* 18–27.

RESTAK, R. M. (1988). *The mind.* New York: Bantam Books.

RILEY, T. L. (1985). Normal sleep patterns. In T. E. Riley (Ed.), *Clinical aspects of sleep and sleep disturbance.* Boston: Butterworth.

ROLLMAN, B., BLOCK, M. R., & SCHULBERG, H. C. (1996). Symptoms of major depression resemble tricyclic side effects. *Psychopharmacology Update, 7*(10), 1–3.

ROSENBAUM, J. F. (1988). The course and treatment of manic-depressive illness: An update. *Journal of Clinical Psychiatry, 49*(11), 3–6.

ROY-BYRNE, P. P. (1992). Integrated treatment of panic disorder. *American Journal of Medicine, 92*(Suppl.), 49S–54S.

SACKEIM, H. A. (1997). Proper ECT dosage optimizes treatment response. *Psychopharmacology Update, 8*(4), 1,5,6.

SAKLAD, S. R. (Ed.). (1997). Benefits of new sustained-release bupropion: Less frequent dosing, fewer side effects. *Psychopharmacology Update, 8*(11), 1,6,7.

SAKLAD, S. R. (Ed.). (1997). News update—suicide. *Psychopharmacology Update, 8*(9), 3.

SAKLAD, S. R. (Ed.). (1997). New antidepressants have advantages over older agents. *Psychopharmacology Update, 8*(10), 1,5,6.

SANDERSON, W. C., & WETZLER, S. (1993). Observations on the cognitive behavioral treatment of panic disorder: Impact of benzodiazepines. *Psychotherapy, 30,* 125–132.

SCHATZBERG, A. F., & COLE, J. O. (1986). *Manual of clinical psychopharmacology.* Washington, DC: American Psychiatric Press.

SHUKLA, A., & COOK, B. L. (1989). Efficacy and safety of lithium-carbamazepine combination in mania. In B. Lerer & S. Gershon (Eds.), *New directions in affective disorders* (pp. 557–562). New York: Springer-Verlag.

SILVERSTONE, T. (1989). Psychopharmacology of schizoaffective mania. In B. Lerer & S. Gershon (Eds.), *New directions in affective disorders* (pp. 495–500). New York: Springer-Verlag.

SIRIS, S. G., BERMANZOHN, P., GONZALEZ, A., MASON, S., WHITE, C., & SHUWALL, M. (1991). The use of antidepressants for negative symptoms in a subset of schizophrenic patients. *Psychopharmacology Bulletin, 27,* 331–335.

SPENCER, E. K., KAFANTARIS, V., PADRON-GAYOL, M. V., ROSENBERG, C. R., & CAMPBELL, M. (1992). Haloperidol in schizophrenic children: Early findings from a study in progress. *Psychopharmacology Bulletin, 28*(2), 183–186.

STAHL, S. M. (1992). The current impact of neuroscience on psychotropic drug discovery and development. *Psychopharmacology Bulletin, 28*(1), 3–9.

STEWART, J. W., QUITKIN, F., & KLEIN, D. (1992). The pharmacotherapy of minor depression. *American Journal of Psychotherapy, 96,* 23–37.

STOUDEMIRE, A. (1995). Expanding psychopharmacologic treatment options for the depressed medical patient. *Psychosomatics, 36*(2), S19–S26.

SUPERNAW, R. B. (1991a). Pharmacotherapeutic management of acute pain. *U.S. Pharmacist,* pp. H-1, 2, 4, 7, 11, 13, 14.

SUPERNAW, R. B. (1991b). Recurrent headache syndromes. *U.S. Pharmacist,* pp. 33, 34, 37, 38, 42, 47, 48, 50, 52, 54.

SWONGER, A. K., & MATEJSKI, M. P. (1991). *Nursing pharmacology.* Philadelphia: Lippincott.

SZEINBACH, S. L., & SUMMERS, K. H. (1992, May). Improving pharmacotherapeutic outcomes in panic disorder. *Drug Topics,* pp. 1–10.

TATRO, D. S., OW-WING, S. D., & HUIE, D. L. (1986). Drug toxicology. In A. M. Pagliaro & L. A. Pagliaro (Eds.), *Pharmacologic aspects of nursing* (pp. 180–187). St. Louis: Mosby.

TAYLOR, R. L. (1990). *Distinguishing psychological from organic disorders.* New York: Springer.

TEST, M. A., BURKE, S. S., & WALLISCH, L. S. (1990). Gender differences of young adults with schizophrenic disorders in community care. *Schizophrenia Bulletin, 16*(2), 331–344.

TEXAS DEPARTMENT OF MENTAL HEALTH AND MENTAL RETARDATION. (1998). Bipolar disorders module: BPD guideline procedures manual. *Texas Medication Algorhythm Project*. Austin, TX: Texas Department of Mental Health and Mental Retardation.

THASE, M. E. (1997). When is psychotherapy alone enough and when is pharmacotherapy better? *Psychopharmacology Update, 8*(4), 1,7.

THOMAS, C. L. (Ed.). (1985). *Taber's cyclopedic medical dictionary* (15th ed.). Philadelphia: Davis.

TORNATORE, F. L. (Ed.). (1996). Know the facts about serotonin syndrome. *Psychopharmacology Update, 7*(11), 1,6.

TRIMBLE, M. R. (1990). Worldwide use of clomipramine. *Journal of Clinical Psychiatry, 51*(8)(Suppl.), 51–54.

TYRER, P. J., & SEIVEWRIGHT, N. (1984). Identification and management of benzodiazepine dependence. *Postgraduate Medical Journal, 60*(2), 41–46.

WALLIS, C., & WILLWERTH, J. (1992, July 6). Schizophrenia: A new drug brings patients back to life. *Time*, pp. 53–60.

WATERMAN, G. S., & RYAN, N. D. (1993). Pharmacological treatment of depression and anxiety in children and adolescents. *School Psychology Review, 22*, 228–242.

WINCOR, M. Z. (1990, January). Sleep disorders. *U.S. Pharmacist, 90*(01), 26, 28–32, 35, 36, 41, 42, 44.

WOOLF, D. S. (1983). CNS depressants. In G. Bennett, C. Vourakis, & D. S. Woolf (Eds.), *Substance abuse*. New York: Wiley.

WRIGHT, C. (1996). Reactions to benzodiazepines. In K. Stovell (Ed.), *Psychotropic medications* (pp. 203–206, 214–217). Providence, RI: Manisses Communications Group, Inc.

YESAVAGE, J. A. (1992). Depression in the elderly. *Postgraduate Medicine, 91*, 255–261.

ZENARDI, R., FRANCHINI, L., GASPERINI, M., & PEREZ, J. (1996). Double-blind controlled trial of sertraline versus paroxetine in the treatment of delusional depression. *American Journal of Psychiatry, 153*, 1631–1633.

ZIEGLER, J. (1997). Benefits parity: What's a healthy mind worth? *Business and Health, 15*(9), 46–57.

MEDICATIONS INDEX

INDEX

TO THE OWNER OF THIS BOOK:

I hope that you have found *Psychotherapist's Resource on Psychiatric Medications* useful. So that this book can be improved in a future edition, would you take the time to complete this sheet and return it? Thank you.

School and address: _____

_____

Department: _____

Instructor's name: _____

1. What I like most about this book is: _____

_____

_____

2. What I like least about this book is: _____

_____

_____

3. My general reaction to this book is: _____

_____

_____

4. The name of the course in which I used this book is: _____

_____

5. Were all of the chapters of the book assigned for you to read?_____

   If not, which ones weren't? _____

6. In the space below, or on a separate sheet of paper, please write specific suggestions for improving this book and anything else you'd care to share about your experience in using this book.

_____

_____

_____

_____

OPTIONAL:

Your name: _____ Date: _____

May we quote you, either in promotion for *Psychotherapist's Resource on Psychiatric Medications*, or in future publishing ventures?

Yes: _____ No: _____

Sincerely yours,

George Buelow
Suzanne Hebert
Sidne Buelow

- -
FOLD HERE

‖‖‖ ‖

NO POSTAGE
NECESSARY
IF MAILED
IN THE
UNITED STATES

BUSINESS REPLY MAIL
FIRST CLASS   PERMIT NO. 358   PACIFIC GROVE, CA

POSTAGE WILL BE PAID BY ADDRESSEE

ATTN: *Counseling Editor, Eileen Murphy*

BROOKS/COLE/THOMSON LEARNING
511 FOREST LODGE ROAD
PACIFIC GROVE, CA   93950-9968

‖‖‖‖‖‖‖‖‖‖‖‖‖‖‖‖‖‖‖‖‖‖‖‖‖‖‖‖‖‖

- -
FOLD HERE